Rethinking
ObeCITY

(Pronounced 'Obese-City')

Doctor Robyn Littlewood

Rethinking
ObeCITY
(Pronounced 'Obese-City')

Krispy Kreme

McDonald's

KFC

Doctor Robyn Littlewood

First Edition 2024

Copyright © 2024 Doctor Robyn Littlewood

National Library of Australia
Cataloguing-in-Publication entry:

Rethinking ObeCITY (Pronounced 'Obese-City') - Doctor Robyn Littlewood

1st ed.
ISBN: 978-1-7635283-0-7 (pbk.)

NATIONAL LIBRARY OF AUSTRALIA   A catalogue record for this book is available from the National Library of Australia

Published by Doctor Robyn Littlewood

Dedication

I would like to dedicate this book to all the beautiful children and families who have trusted me to support their medical and nutritional health and wellbeing over the past few decades. I have walked into so many waiting rooms feeling relentlessly optimistic for the future of these beautiful Queenslanders, who, along with their families, had clearly lost hope a long time ago. When focusing on each child and their family, all I could see was the enormous potential they couldn't even imagine was true. Why? Their environment didn't support them. In fact, the conditions in their lives were making it so difficult, they couldn't try anymore. Their 'village' had been taken away from them. These kids and their families were ceasing to thrive in a way that all children should and have been able to in the past.

In my view, their surroundings and the external factors that made up those surrounds were influencing them in a negative way. There was limited ability for young, creative minds to consider the way they could change and influence their environment back, or even if they could at all. There was a real shortage of resources, support

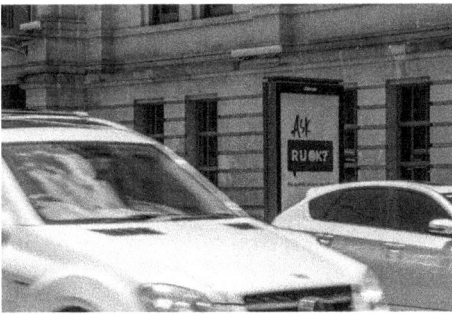

and guidance to help people create a village full of hope and real happiness. I feel this is missing today. Nobody was throwing them a lifeline or giving these children the real facts, despite being the most well-intentioned, loving and adoring parents, families, friends and health professionals. These children and their families, along with the health services and communities supporting them, had lost their way and the environment was reinforcing that.

At the end of every consultation, my main goal was to ensure two things:

- Firstly, that these beautiful families understood their surrounding system; an environment that was not working to support them, in fact, more likely it was working against them. Sadly, the extent of the challenges is often based on where they lived. Usually, the most vulnerable communities and regions have the harshest influences.

- Secondly, that they understood their true potential and how they could push back to build, grow and thrive. I wanted them to believe in their ability to influence their surroundings. They needed to question, to seek alternatives and the truth about their environment. I wanted them to know how to do this well and sustainably to set them up for a better life. A life of choice; not chance.

To achieve a better life, we need help. We can't do something that big and important on our own. Understanding that is the first step to improving outcomes. We all need an environment that supports us to be creative, motivated, happy and supportive of our health and wellbeing. It's only when we achieve this, that our 'place' stops influencing us as a city, but rather, supports us as 'our village'. This is the space that surrounds us including where we grow, live, work, play and sleep. It's the place that influences all that we do but in a positive, connected, and supportive way. That's what a village means to me. Our city is making decisions for us. It is telling us what to buy, how much to spend, how to move, what to cook, when to sleep, what to watch and often, how to feel. Our village is different and this is what I want for everyone.

What if…

- Healthy meals were cheaper than hot chips; would we eat healthy foods more?

- School ovals were more accessible and open on weekends; would we use them more?

- Bikes were available and bike paths were completed and connected across all parts of our community; would we cycle more?

- We all had cooking skills to make easy, affordable and healthy dinners and the time to do it; would we cook more?

- What if we weren't bullied at school or we knew the way to manage bullying well if we were; would our kids feel less anxious about going to school?

- What if food labels were easier to read and actually said what they meant; would we make different choices as we could read and understand the labelling better?

- What if we didn't feel guilt or shame about our weight or our health and were able to talk more openly to our loving families and professionals when we needed to, about what was important to us; would our most vulnerable people and loved ones feel more connected and engaged in the community?

- What if we all knew how to get help when we needed it and knew who to talk to when our mental health was compromised; would we access help more?

I would guess that some, if not most of your answers to these questions above are **yes.** It is definitely the vision I have for my family - 'my village'. This is exactly what I want you to create for yours. What if I told you this was all possible? Life needs to be about choice and opportunity, to help us be healthy and happy. None of our outcomes should be up to chance (i.e. where we live, our postcode or our region). We can achieve it all, but we need to be empowered to do so.

Life is also different for many of us, as we don't all start from the same place. That's why the things we need to understand and influence, will be different for different environments, different suburbs and even different streets in the same suburb. Our villages will look different, but will perform the same function – to empower, to support and to believe.

I remember every single child walking into my waiting room. With eyes looking down, avoiding any engagement. All I could ever see were children and families, so affected by their current situation, feeling so guilty and ashamed of the outcomes; being that of increased weight and poor physical, emotional, mental or social health. They had no idea that none of this was their fault and completely out of their control and the weight of guilt hung over their head, heavy and debilitating. The stigma and consistent shameful messaging had taken its toll.

They had no idea how important they truly were, and how much they inspired me every day. I felt compelled to write a book about them. They *are* the reason I can do my job with the laser-focus I need every day to lead, empower and believe. It should never be up to chance to decide what children have in life but rather, they all need to believe in change with choice. You also need the tools to do it. This includes the facts, as difficult as they can be to understand.

By chance, I mean we are all born into different families, homes and communities, however, that should never define our outcomes. With hope comes change and this is where I want to position the beautiful next generation of Queensland children; to believe in themselves, not in the pre-determined version, according to where they were born.

A couple of messages I want you to be completely clear about:

1. If things are tough and you feel you have little control, you are probably completely right, but you CAN do something and the time is right to start.
2. The environment around you is modifiable - you just need to understand it and you can change it. It will be a journey, but worth it.
3. Question the previous and the status quo. Just because it's always been that way, doesn't mean it has to continue.
4. You are definitely worth it.

5. You have the right to good health.
6. Your future is not what your environment reinforces to you. In fact, it's often the opposite.
7. You need your village. It's possible and it's time to build it again.
8. It's the right time to do it.

Finally, I also want to dedicate this book to my beautiful father who has worked hard through some very significant personal health challenges. Following a simple fall leading to enduring more than 30 spinal surgeries, resulting in a diagnosis of incomplete quadriplegia, my dad remains positive and motivated. He has empowered me and believed in my work throughout the many university years, degrees and qualifications and through my work at Health and Wellbeing Queensland. He wears a Health and Wellbeing Queensland hat and shirt most days and 'wheels' through our physical activity challenges. He takes what life throws at him and turns it into days filled with humour and dignity. He has continued to empower and believe in me and my work and is my greatest fan. He created 'my village'. Don't ever underestimate the influence you have on your children. You continue to guide them, influence them and shape their thinking, often at times when you don't think they're listening at all. It is so powerful.

I hope reading this will help inspire more people to understand their surroundings and how to push back on it when needed and how to create surroundings that are good, supportive and hopeful. Once you do that, you will have started to create a village and this is when you can thrive.

Dedication

We all want the best for our children. I hope this book helps, even a little, to remind you how you and they can do exactly that - thrive. It's a hard environment. You know that. It's time to know that the environment doesn't have to decide for you, what you will do and become. You can do that, when supported by your village. We all need one! Here's a little 'how-to' guide on how to create a better place, a better village, a better city, no matter who you are or where you live.

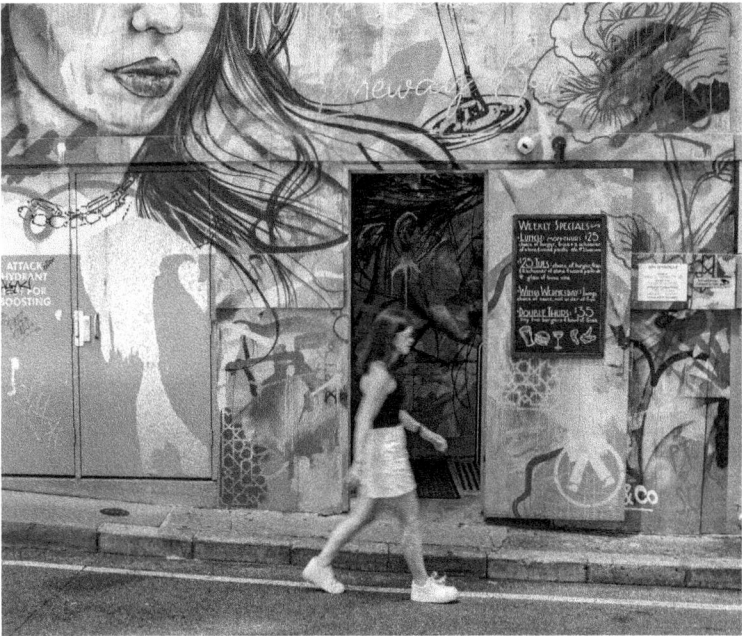

Table of contents

Foreword

There is an old saying that it is better to light a candle than to curse the darkness. In health terms, we live in a darkening world. Several experts in different countries have warned that young people today have a shorter life expectancy than their parents. A whole series of pressures have been driving people to make poor choices about food and drink, about physical exercise, about legal and illegal drugs, about screen time, about social groups. The organisations which get rich on the proceeds have unleashed a flood of carefully orchestrated misinformation to persuade us to make those poor choices. We desperately need a light to guide us through those misleading advertisements and social pressures to help us make wise choices. Our health and that of our children is at stake.

This book is better than a candle. It is a bright, shining light. Dr Robyn Littlewood has a long and distinguished career in the health care sector, predominantly helping children and their parents to keep the young ones healthy. A few years ago, she was appointed to head a new government agency, Health and Wellbeing Queensland. Under her leadership, the agency has a wide range of programs designed to improve the health of Queenslanders, especially children and young adults who live in traditionally disadvantaged areas. She understands that the best thing we can do to help our young people stay healthy is show them how to avoid practices that lead to poor outcomes later in life. This important book is based on her decades of experience, her accumulated wisdom and her passionate belief that we can transform the practices that are making us less healthy.

As you read this book, you will be startled by the hard evidence that shows how we have steadily become less healthy. Then you will be cheered up by the remedies Dr Littlewood explains. It is important to remember that the future is not somewhere we are going. It is something we are creating. There isn't one inevitable pre-determined future. There are many possible futures. Which one happens will be determined by the choices we all make: as individuals, members of families, members of communities and organisations. Just as the City has been making us unwell, this book explains how we can develop Villages that keep us healthy. Where you live influences your choices. Whether you are in a city, a town or a remote area shapes many of your options: whether healthy food and drink are available and affordable, what open space you have for exercise and recreation, what access you have to natural areas, what social factors help or hinder your path to good health. There isn't a single prescription that you can follow, wherever you live in this vast and diverse State. But there are general principles that can help you to take advantage of where you live, to steer away from unhealthy practices, to celebrate the good aspects of your surroundings. This is your guidebook for that journey.

Emeritus Professor Ian Lowe
Widely published and highly awarded expert on urban development, sustainability, environmental science and public health

Introduction – ObeCITY vs village?

Globally right now, regardless of where we live, our city is making us sick. Our environment influences how we eat, move, sleep, play and work. It is deliberate, manipulative, and highly effective. The 'health' food industry and fitness sectors are thriving, yet the health of our population is getting worse.

The following facts are commonly known. Obesity rates are increasing. Chronic disease rates are increasing and the rates of people feeling mentally and physically unwell are increasing. In the 1970s, when I was at school, overweight and obesity rates for children were 1-2 per cent. That is, one or two children per 100 were living with overweight or obesity. Today, in Australia, this number is closer to one in four children, and this keeps me up at night. The changes I see emerging from my generation to my children's are clear. Life has become less tolerant, more impatient, faster paced, and even more judgemental. The demands of our cities and our systems on our families to ensure success at work, school and healthcare have increased globally and as such, our cities have become much less personalised, more complicated and challenging to navigate. It is so easy to feel lost more than ever before. As we all do our best to navigate this new world of complexity, it's no wonder our overall health is starting to decline with obesity rates increasing. What's more worrying is the future years for our children. We are all accountable to the next generation and as such, I feel compelled to do something about it. Writing this book is hopefully just one small positive contribution.

Nobody likes the word 'obesity'. The use of the word is currently subject to considerable controversy. Throughout my long career of presenting on the topic of obesity, health, paediatrics and research, the debate of whether to use the term obesity compared to other terms such as 'living in a larger body' arises and, in my opinion, takes up way too much time and energy. I have always lived by a few basic principles regarding obesity within my clinics and they have steered me well. I would like to share them with you and explain the use of the word obesity throughout this book.

1. Use obesity to describe a medical condition.
2. Don't bother giving the use of the word 'obesity' oxygen or media attention by debating the use. The debate is a distraction from the real work that needs to be done.
3. Use the term accurately and sensitively. This will ensure you can't go wrong.
4. Weight stigma is real and should never be tolerated in any form. The effects can be devastating and pervasive.
5. ObeCITY accurately implies an external reason for the increase in obesity rates. There should be no judgement or blame to any individual, ever. This includes if people choose to be happy in their own body, regardless of size, shape or weight. This book isn't about the use of the term 'obesity'. Rather, it's about everything else.
6. Always use the term 'village' to describe where someone lives when improving their environment. A village is a lovely, positive inference of place that you can mould, shape and build on. In fact, if you create 'your village' well, you won't have to worry about the other five principles.

Life is hard and currently, it's getting harder. There are lots of barriers out there which hold negative obstacles and their consequences in place. We need to build a defence – a loving, supportive, friendly, kind and empowering frontline of protection.

I want to start this book by validating what you've all been thinking and feeling for the past years. The current environment has changed and yes, it is really hard. Some of the issues you are experiencing are the same for many of us and shared across all parts of Queensland and Australia. Some may be unique to you or you might be hearing some of this for the first time. Knowing and understanding issues that surround us is critical for change to occur.

If you are finding times are tougher to navigate, you'd be right.
If you are finding times are much more challenging financially and the cost of living is so much higher, you'd be right.

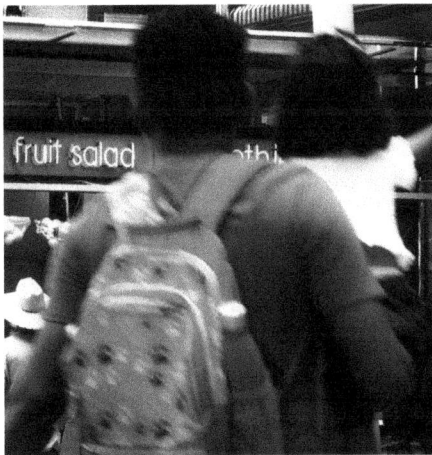

If you feel the stress of providing a healthy diet, supportive environment and community for your children as they grow, for your family or just for yourself, you should know that current anxiety rates and feelings of depression are actually increasing. In Queensland, one in two adults are concerned about their wellbeing, yet 40 per cent of us feel we can't do anything about it. This is why our health is not improving. We are stuck, but there is a way out of it.

The year 2020 was something new. It was hard but it had a feeling of uniqueness to it. We used the word 'pivot' a lot more and were busy trying to cope with what the pandemic meant for each of us individually, and that was very different for all of us. Some of us lost our jobs, some of us were locked up tight in our communities. Some worked from home, some worked double shifts on the frontline in healthcare and some found it hard to keep stock on shelves in supermarkets. This time was uncertain and we navigated all of it as best we could. However, we also started to question the status quo which is what I still believe is the complete silver lining that came from COVID-19.

The year 2021 was supposed to be better.

Some of us gained more weight without trying. Some of us lost weight out of worry.

Some of us became the healthiest we had ever been.

Some of us joined the big 'walkout movement', leaving their jobs in search of a better work-life balance. Some of us were infected by COVID-19 and became really sick and are still struggling with some of the effects to our health.

Suicide attempts increased and suicide rates sadly also increased. Sport participation declined and people felt out of control of their lives.

The research showed many of us lost motivation. It was at this point, many of my patients would tell me it was their fault that they were feeling lazy, in which case, I would always correct them. The feeling of being overwhelmed and immobilised by the uncertainty, was completely out of their control. It wasn't about being lazy at all.

Then, 2022 was something else. It was more of the same but somehow it felt harder. It has been about adjusting to the 'new norm'. It was about recovering, however, many of us were unsure what we were recovering from whilst many reported this ongoing sense of lack of motivation and connection.

I want to provide a sense of clarity for you. This is the most critical message in the whole book. If you don't read on, please understand this paragraph. To truly improve your health, you need to understand the barriers you are dealing with, which probably wasn't what you were thinking or expecting. It's not your fault that you're feeling tired and it's definitely not that you're too lazy to get back into life. However, I don't want you to think that you can't make change and you can't take control. You absolutely can, but you have to know how.

Our city is determining our health, in fact, it's making us sick. Building a village will keep us well.

City, can be defined as a relatively permanent and highly organised centre of a population, of greater size or importance than a town. In my opinion, it is where environmental factors often dominate and influence people by chance, without warning or awareness. In other words, if you're born into a city or region, the environment will want to already pre-determine lots of your outcomes, without you being aware of it.

A village is described as "community life, where you know every one of the people you live around". It is also a place that empowers people to choose their destination, by understanding the choices offered and the decisions to accept or reject their influences. This is where you create 'your village' and take control back in your life.

This goal of this book will help you shift from living in a city to a living in a village, without you moving locations. It's about creating the village in the city you live in. It is definitely possible.

We need a village to remind us that life doesn't have to be as hard as it is. Starting the journey to create your village will be hard. Starting to question your environment, refusing to go with the flow and pushing back will take time and effort. However, it is worth getting it right for the rest of your life, but it will be exhausting at the start.

COVID-19 is important to truly understand. It didn't cause the effects on our environment, however, it certainly made the impact the environment has on us so much more visible to us all. Using the

COVID-19 period as an example to demonstrate why your village is so important, is an easier way to describe the social determinants of health and why getting this right within our village is critical. It is also a perfect demonstration of the effects of inequity and how this caused such cumulative damage in our cities or regions.

In my opinion, 2023 was harder again. It seemed to be filled with common stories of widening inequities and divides in communities. I see a much greater impact from the increased cost of living for all of us and the implications of that. There has been a plethora of media dominating the news across the country on youth violence and justice and how this has all just emerged.

2024 is already filled with natural disasters and warfare. It seems every country, every state or region has an emergent issue which appears to be worse than the year before. All of these events have an impact on our environment. Specifically in Australia, droughts, rain, flooding, bushfires and cyclones are increasing our cost of living (and that includes 2024). The cost of growing, farming and freighting fresh fruit and vegetables is increasing at a time where our communities are still recovering from the previous disasters. Our feeling of food security, and even personal safety in our communities, is the most fragile I can remember.

This all hasn't just emerged. We have been in the middle of a perfect storm for some time now. I hope my book explains a little more to those who have polarised views on today's challenges. Creating a long-term sustainable village, rather than building overnight cities or regions full of anger and trauma, is much more effective in changing the trajectory of lives for the next generation of children. I want to explain to you why and give you the evidence so you can make up your own mind.

Our children and our children's children are depending on it.

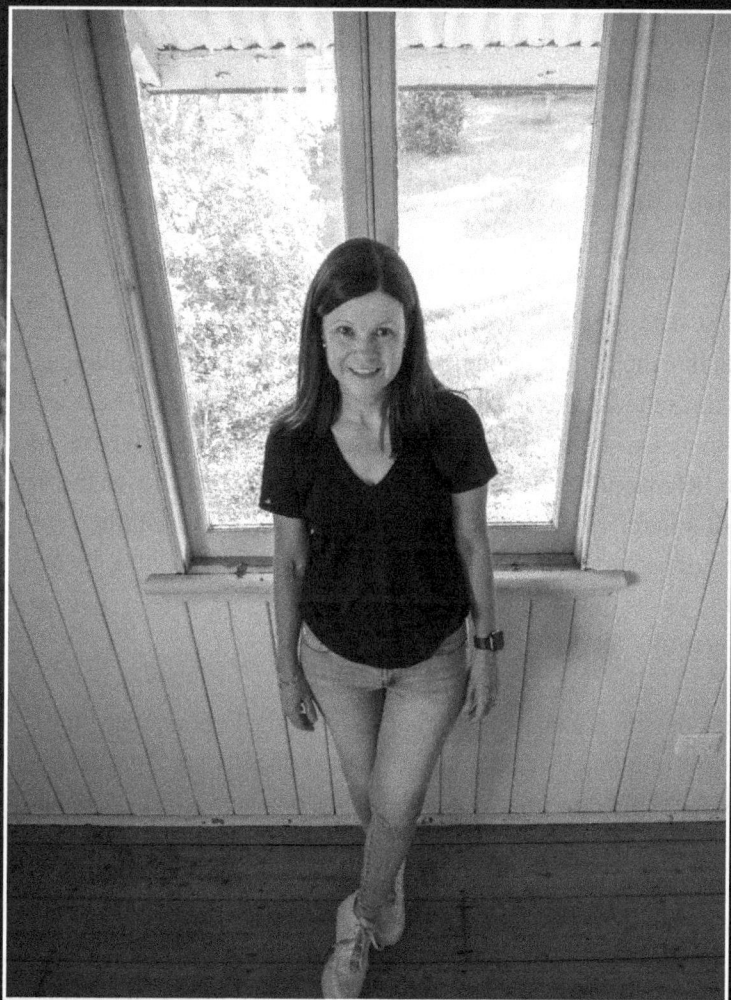

CHAPTER 1

The social determinants of health

CHAPTER 1

The social determinants of health

We know that the things that sit outside of health, affect our health the most, often without us even knowing it. We think these barriers are insignificant and even 'white noise', but they're not. They're working hard against us and maintaining those negative forces every single day. The social conditions that make up where we live, affect us so much. There are determinants that impact and shape these conditions.

Social determinants are factors that make up where you live, including the food environment, access to education, cost of living, housing, and access to green space, just to name a few. These are the things you can't control but have an incredible influence on your behaviour. You can certainly push back on and change these, but it's hard. Understanding what they are and the simple steps you can take to influence your own environment is helpful. I want you to understand exactly what they are for you, as they will be different for all of us.

These determinants are hard enough to navigate in regular times. However, in times of devastation, natural disasters or a pandemic, these social determinants double down on their impact – either in a negative or positive way. This is what COVID-19 did to us. This is a perfect example of inequities and how this worsened inconsistently throughout the pandemic.

For example:

If we used to run daily, exercise and eat healthy prior to COVID-19, through COVID-19 we probably did this more. In fact, we signed up for the first time to exercise apps and counted our steps. We bought new exercise gear and walked the dog, over and over again.

Alternatively, if we didn't exercise prior to COVID-19, we probably found exercise even more challenging and out of reach. Our weight was often affected as a result.

Prior to COVID-19, if we provided healthy food daily to our families, we continued this through COVID-19 with more of an emphasis on healthy foods, baking and cooking options. Alternatively, if prior to 2019, we found healthy food expensive and hard to find, food became more out of reach, less accessible and even more expensive throughout the pandemic. Our weight was affected as a result.

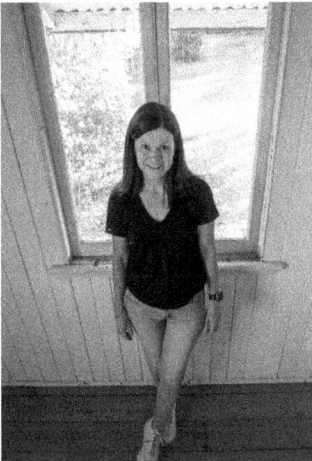

What's happening is that the environment is deciding what is going to be accessible to you, what's going to be challenging and the panic from a pandemic will always amplify these outcomes. It's all the things around you, the social determinants, that continue either to support you or challenge you, and they become so much stronger and even more polarising in their impact in times of uncertainty.

The remainder of this chapter will demonstrate to you how hard the environment has become in Australia. There is SO MUCH influence affecting you, providing you with little choice and options. Unless you understand these forces, it will be very difficult for you to change but you must remember that you can control them. You just need to know what they are.

In the current environment, I don't know how anyone is actually able to maintain a healthy lifestyle and a healthy weight. I have to work at ensuring my health and wellbeing is good, day in and day out. It's not easy but I make a conscious effort every day.

When wondering how to explain the way to build your supportive environment, 'your village', you must truly understand it. Read any newspaper, watch any mainstream morning news program, or listen to any mainstream radio station and you will see the same gap I do. Where are the credible facts and figures showing us what's going on in our environment? If you wander through the sensational headlines and infomercials, what's at the core of this information? Is it factual or not?

COVID-19 confirmed for me something I already knew. People want the facts and figures to make their own deductions. Our population is mature, sophisticated, and analytical and can more easily make sense of their own surroundings if provided with accurate, relevant and credible information. You don't need others around you making assumptions for you.

Despite this, it's still not commonplace to find a list of facts and figures about what has changed in the environment. Some would say, this would be more appropriately positioned within an academic journal article or research paper. However, in my opinion, this is what is missing in Australia right now across almost all media - the facts.

People believe it is their fault that things are becoming more difficult and complicated as this is often what the messaging is telling them and clearly, what they're hearing. This is evident in increased suicide rates and demand for mental health services for many more of us. I want to reassure you, with words and statistics, that this is not the case. Hence, this book is about to get a little boring and quite heavy, but I think it's the critical part. To understand the truth, you must understand why you feel the way you do. Best of all, by truly understanding the changes in the current environment, you will also understand how to make changes. That's what this journey is all about, for all of us. After this chapter, you will understand what the social determinants of health are and how they truly play a role in our lives.

Please stick with the facts and figures. It may support you to feel a complete sense of relief. "This isn't actually my fault and it's not just me". You may also feel completely validated in your thinking and feeling. I am hoping you will feel empowered when you are reassured that you are not alone and people around you are feeling exactly the same way as you are. This can, and will, help motivate you to do something about it.

Below are some social factors that I believe are having a huge impact on our lives. There are many more, however, these are very relevant to our health and wellbeing journey. I will explain further as we work our way through this book.

1. **The increasing population** - the estimated resident Queensland population in 2022 was 5,326,622 people.[1] The most populated Queensland areas in 2021 were major cities (64.8%), followed by inner regional (19.4%), outer regional (13.4%), remote (1.4%) and very remote (1.0%).[1] This is important to understand for many reasons. Where we live affects our health, with the level of remoteness impacting it directly, i.e., the more remote your location the more negatively your health is impacted.

The population of Queensland is projected to increase by 2042, a further 34 per cent from the 2022 figure, meaning there will be more than 7 million people in the state.[2] From these numbers, the social condition of housing or finding accommodation will become more and more at risk. To afford a house, to pay the rent and keep up with rental increases, is often unattainable now. With increases in population and demand, this will only continue to worsen as people continue to move to regional and remote areas in search of a house they can afford. With such a housing crisis emerging, cost of living will also increase. Challenges will ensue, to create new pressures and obstacles in our lives. This impacts our health and wellbeing significantly and in so many ways.

2. **The increasing cost of living** - in 2023-2024 in Australia, this has been leading news for months and is about to get even worse. Easing cost of living was the focus of the Federal Budget for 2022-23 and 2023-24, and I suspect for several years to come. It was proposed that the one-off $250 welfare

payment and the $420 increase in the temporary low- and middle-income tax offset, would help many families tie ends together which is on the right track.[3] However, as good as increases were, they have been quickly outweighed by escalating household costs.

We know that in Australia, anyone relying on Centrelink benefits to survive must spend approximately half of their income to purchase food that is healthy to feed their family. This has always been so much worse for those living in rural and regional areas, with the acceptance of 'the more remote, the higher the cost' due to freight, weather, distance and access issues. In Queensland, this is particularly bad as the level of remoteness and isolation is high. These outcomes are even worse.

"Healthy diets cost 34 per cent more in very remote areas of Queensland than in Brisbane, and a whopping 41 per cent more in the Torres Strait Islands".[3]

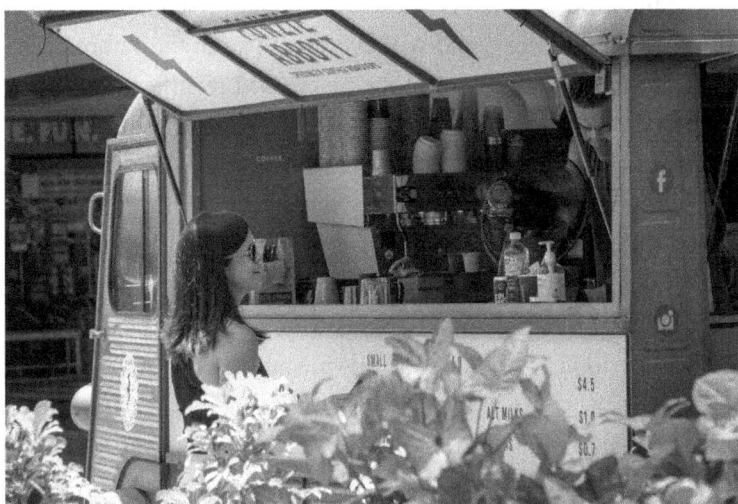

I have recently learned that one in three homes in some of the most remote areas of far north Queensland don't have enough food to last one day. Food insecurity is a significant problem in Queensland and other parts of the country, yet many Australians are not aware of the extent of the issue and how it's impacting their neighbours.

"Food prices are increasing due to rising fuel, feed and fertiliser costs, and disruptions to local and global food production and supply due to COVID-19, climate change and extreme weather events, and now the impacts of the Russian invasion of Ukraine".[3]

Supermarkets continue to advertise their attempts at keeping prices stable, however, anyone who does their household shopping is well-aware of the increase that is evident for just about every product. This comes on the back of significant increases to the price of most healthy foods during the COVID-19 pandemic, shown in recent studies in Queensland. As prices of healthy food are driven upwards, unhealthy ultra-processed foods have become relatively cheaper. Consequently, many families are consuming less healthy diets, which is already having adverse health impacts (those 'COVID kilos') and will even more so in the future. "The price of most healthy food groups increased significantly during the pandemic—with the exception of some canned vegetables and legumes, which decreased".[4] Conversely, the price of discretionary foods (those filled with fat and sugar) and sugary drinks, did not increase during the pandemic.[4] The cost of providing groceries and food significantly increased throughout this period except for discretionary foods, which continued to be less expensive than the healthy food.[4] In real terms, this meant we bought more foods higher in salt, sugar and fat. The same economic reality caused us to buy less fresh fruit and vegies. Clearly, our communities had little choice. Accessibility doesn't just refer to freight and supply chain issues and position in a supermarket, it also means access through cost. If healthy food is cost prohibitive, families don't have a choice. They buy what they can afford. This is the conundrum. We have no choice!

Whenever I talk about my frustration with the number of fast-food restaurants being approved in Australia, people always remind me that "Australians will always make their own decisions as long as they have choice". In fact, some of the fast-food chain leaders have publicly supported that people want choice and all they are doing is giving it to them. They don't admit they are also happy to make a profit in this situation. I find that unethical or dishonest and here's why.

In more vulnerable areas in Australia (i.e. communities where families survive on fixed means and income), there are more fast-food take away restaurants per capita than regions with higher incomes. This is not a coincidence. The combination of many accessible fast-food restaurants with drive through access and relentless marketing of low-priced meals (one example - five products for $5) encourages us to purchase. Our children will not go to bed hungry, and we will be able to pay our bills at the same time. Now compare this with going to the local supermarket, purchasing fruit and vegies, fresh meat and bread to prepare meals. This cost can be double, unaffordable to many and often forces a decision between paying bills vs providing a healthy meal. Parents will do anything to avoid their children from going hungry. The choice has been taken away from the community, without the community even knowing it. In other words, you don't have choice. Trust me. The companies know it. The marketing giants of the fast-food industry know it and they are banking on it, literally.

Let's look at what happened during COVID-19. Income supplements were paid to Australians during the first stage of the COVID-19 pandemic (May – September 2020). "The affordability of the recommended diet improved greatly, by 27 per cent and 42 per cent, for households with minimum-wage and welfare-only disposable household income, respectively".[4] I am very convinced, when people have enough money, they will buy what's healthy. When they have a choice, they will purchase fruit and vegies for their kids when they can. People enjoy having a choice and they choose well when they do. However, when the choice is removed through access issues such as cost, we will do anything to keep food insecurity away from our children. Buying cheap, often fried, less nutritious take-away meals helps (in the worst sense of the word) us do that.

3. **Increasing domestic violence** – It will be of no surprise to anyone that the pressures experienced within environments and communities from the impact of COVID-19, are having a lasting impact. The feeling of being overwhelmed and unable to mobilise is also manifesting into other major social issues. A study by the Australian Institute of Criminology (AIC) of 15,000 women found increases in domestic violence experienced by Australian women during the first three months of the pandemic.[5] Of these women, two-thirds said that domestic violence had either escalated or started during

the COVID-19 pandemic.[5] Further, it is well accepted that much of this is not reported to the police, so the numbers are probably worse than what we are aware of.

"At the other end of the spectrum, by the end of April 2020, as people were staying home more, rates of common, serious, and sexual assault had declined to their lowest level in a number of years".[6] To be clear, what declined was external, random violence within the community. I can also recall the number of admissions to hospital due to car accidents, injuries from alcohol-related fights, drink driving and late-night social events at bars and parties, had hit an all-time low. Social distancing regulations saw reductions in this type of violent crime. "Social distancing is likely to have significantly limited interpersonal interaction, especially in locations and at times when violence is usually prevalent".[6] This was a silver lining at the time.

However, this was not the case with domestic violence towards women, according to the Queensland Police Service administrative data. This was equally experienced nationally and globally.

While one-in-three women will experience violence during their lifetime, being locked down with violent partners, has increased domestic and family violence (DFV) by more than 25 per cent with some countries reporting rates of DFV doubling.[7]

This is relevant to the discussion on social determinants as the impact of COVID-19 lockdowns and restrictions on those who experienced DFV, affected those who already experienced greater vulnerability, either due to regions of vulnerability, lower socioeconomic status (SES), higher areas of remoteness and just being female.

The groups experiencing vulnerability identified by service providers will not surprise you. They included female clients with school-age children (63%), clients from culturally and linguistically diverse (CALD) communities (47%), female clients with existing domestic violence protection orders (43%) and clients with disabilities (40%,).[8] One-third of service providers reported that COVID-19 had particularly affected clients from rural and remote communities (33%), clients of Aboriginal and/ or Torres Strait Islander descent (32%), and clients in LGBTIQ+ relationships (10%).[8]

If support required face-to-face contact and personalised screening, lockdown made that almost impossible. The previous monitoring offered to groups through regular contact in schools, workplaces and social events, was ceased overnight. Previously, teachers could eyeball children they were worried about every day. With COVID-19, that wasn't possible anymore. Those who were most vulnerable were placed at huge risk because they became almost invisible to the rest of society.

In other parts of the world, violence against women during the COVID-19 pandemic was called the shadow pandemic and was also reported in the most vulnerable areas of inequity.

Again, we all don't start from the same place and where we live so often determines our risk of vulnerability. However, by understanding this, you have the knowledge to know this is not your fault, it's not definitive and you can influence change.

4. **Increased unemployment** – The beginning of the COVID-19 pandemic in 2020 reported a 5.4 per cent decline in employment rates in one month.[9] Outback Queenslanders had the highest unemployment rate at 12.9 per cent, with the overall Queensland unemployment rate sitting at 7.3 per cent within six months.[10] Compared to all respondents, 20 per cent more Queenslanders had their working hours reduced or lost employment due to COVID-19.[10] Across all survey respondents, households experienced a 37 per cent reduction in household income.[10] Twenty-five percent more Queenslanders indicated they had drawn down on their superannuation, in comparison to all respondents.[10] Overall, the impact on all Queenslanders was high, but again, the highest impact was felt by those experiencing greater vulnerability prior to the pandemic.

Among those in casual or part-time work, 46 per cent had a reduction in household income. Of Queensland respondents who were self-employed, 92 per cent were forced to reduce their working or business hours due to COVID-19.[10] Employment changes were substantial for many people during the COVID-19 pandemic, including loss of jobs and businesses, even with substantial mitigation via government support programs (particularly earlier in the pandemic), such as JobKeeper and increases to JobSeeker.[11]

There was a steep decline in average income experienced at the start of the pandemic, with those working in entertainment, hospitality and tourism most starkly affected. Nobody was travelling and it was too 'risky' to go out for dinner! Women were overrepresented as casual employees in industries significantly affected by COVID-19, such as retail (61%) and accommodation and hospitality (54%),[10] so of course, they were the most significantly affected.

In fact, in my opinion, the impact of the pandemic on women will be felt for years to come. Some of the reported impacts so far include:

- The amount of unpaid work increased for women as they reported more responsibility for the entire family through this period.

- More women left the workforce as a result.

- The proportion of women aged 18-54 years who had their working hours cut were overrepresented in comparison to men.

- A greater proportion of women drew down on their superannuation.

- A greater proportion of women reported being kept up at night worrying about paying the bills.

- Women's mental health and wellbeing was more impacted than men.

Does that sound familiar to you? Again, most of this is completely out of our control, but is so important to understand and feel validated that others were feeling this too.

5. **Impacted rates of exercise** – During the pandemic, based on self-reported data conducted by the Australian Bureau of Statistics (ABS) in June 2020, "20.5 per cent of people aged 18 or over increased their time spent on exercise or other physical activity compared to before the pandemic, while 19.2 per cent decreased it".[11] This also confirmed the impacts of inequities mentioned earlier. It appears that if you exercised previously, you were more likely to increase this during the pandemic. If you didn't, again, you doubled down on not doing it. However, there is some good news in more recent times for many of us, particularly women. Studies show an increase in exercise and physical activity levels among adults across the nation and this effect remains[11]. The Australian Sports Commission reported similar outcomes with males returning to their previous sporting levels, however, it was their data on female participation that was surprising. Women reported higher levels of participation than pre-COVID. It is the type of physical activity that appears to be gender specific, with more males participating in team or organised sports and women preferring activities of convenience such as walking. Something good is happening in the environment to support this anomaly for women. Whatever it is, we need more of it.

Put simply, these statistics are close to home, personal and real. They clearly show:

1. Some conditions were already impacting our health prior to COVID-19.

2. If you had any of the issues above, COVID-19 has increased the risk and impact of these conditions, which affected your health even further.

3. There is simply no reference here to personal responsibility. It is very hard to change behaviour without influencing the conditions that support the behaviours in the first place.

4. The barriers that hold inequities in place become negatively supercharged in any disaster. A pandemic is no different.

5. Women are affected and will be for a long time, however, physical activity appears to be improving.

WHAT THIS MEANS FOR YOUR VILLAGE:
We've all just been doing what we've been told.

I hope the heaviness of this chapter has also provided you with a better understanding of what's been happening. It's a perfect storm. Life is hard, but it's also possible to make a difference, now that you know what's really going on.

Chapter 1 References
1. Department of Housing and Public Works. 2023. *Queensland Housing Profiles – dwelling and household characteristics, Queensland* [Online]. Queensland Government. Available: https://statistics.qgso.qld.gov.au/profiles/hpw/housing/pdf/45GDHLQXHD202HNVA6QG-E217OEO692F1K3Q56UO94R2P2R-7JK0VF7T6SJ4JQO5Z2HT58BC5FXT-6GT8R8EJLHVMU48AWUZNBLK8YE-3CYHT1V11X1YO58JRT6P322B0G0I/hpw-housing-profiles#view=fit&pagemode=bookmarks [Accessed 2023].
2. Queensland Government Statistician's Office. 2018. *Queensland Government population projects* [Online]. Queensland Treasury. Available: https://www.qgso.qld.gov.au/issues/2671/qld-government-population-projections-2018-edn.pdf [Accessed 2023].
3. Lee, A., Herron, LM. & Fredericks, B. 7 April 2022. As we face a "perfect storm" for food security, here are some solutions. Available from: https://medicine.uq.edu.au/blog/2022/04/we-face-%E2%80%9Cperfect-storm%E2%80%9D-food-security-here-are-some-solutions 2023].
4. Lee, A. J., Patay, D., Herron, L.-M., Tan, R. C., Nicoll, E., Fredericks, B. & Lewis, M. 2021. Affordability of Heathy, Equitable and More Sustainable Diets in Low-Income Households in Brisbane before and during the COVID-19 Pandemic. *Nutrients* [Online], 13.
5. Carrington, K., Morley, C., Warren, S., Ryan, V., Ball, M., Clarke, J. & Vitis, L. 2021. The impact of COVID-19 pandemic on Australian domestic and family violence services and their clients. *Australian Journal of Social Issues,* 56**,** 539-558.
6. Payne, J. L., Morgan, A. & Piquero, A. R. 2022. COVID-19 and social distancing measures in Queensland, Australia, are associated with short-term decreases in recorded violent crime. *Journal of Experimental Criminology,* 18**,** 89-113.

7. Queensland Government Statistician's Office. 2021. *COV-ID-19 and DFV assault offence trends, March–September 2020.* [Online]. Queensland Treasury. Available: https://www.qgso.qld.gov.au/issues/11116/covid-19-dfv-assault-offence-trends-march-september-2020.pdf [Accessed 2023].

8. Morley, C., Carrington, K., Ryan, V., Warren, S., Clarke, J., Ball, M. & Vitis, L. 2021. Locked Down with the Perpetrator: The Hidden Impacts of COVID-19 on Domestic and Family Violence in Australia. *International Journal for Crime, Justice and Social Democracy,* 10, 204-222.

9. Queensland Treasury. 2023. *Queensland Government Statistician's Office – Labour and employment.* [Online]. Queensland Government. Available: https://www.qgso.qld.gov.au/statistics/theme/economy/labour-employment/state [Accessed 2023].

10. Queensland Council of Social Service. 2020. *COVID-19 impacts on Queenslanders. The unfolding impacts of COVID-19 and how they are distributed among different people.* [Online]. Available: https://www.qcoss.org.au/wp-content/uploads/2021/02/QCOSS-Queensland-Impacts-COVID-19.pdf [Accessed 2023].

11. Australian Institute of Health and Welfare. 2022. *Australia's health 2022 – data insights: Changes in the health of Australians during the COVID-19 period.* [Online]. Available: https://www.aihw.gov.au/getmedia/cb5f5bbb-df0b-4a1c-9796-25ea2e94e447/aihw-aus-240_Chapter_2.pdf.aspx [Accessed 2023].

12. Australian Sports Commission. 2021. AusPlay Focus - Ongoing impact of COVID-19 on sport and physical activity participation June 2021 update. Australian Government. Available: https://www.clearinghouseforsport.gov.au/__data/assets/pdf_file/0004/1012846/AusPlay-COVID-19-update-June-2021.pdf [Accessed 2024]

CHAPTER 2

Is our health actually getting worse?

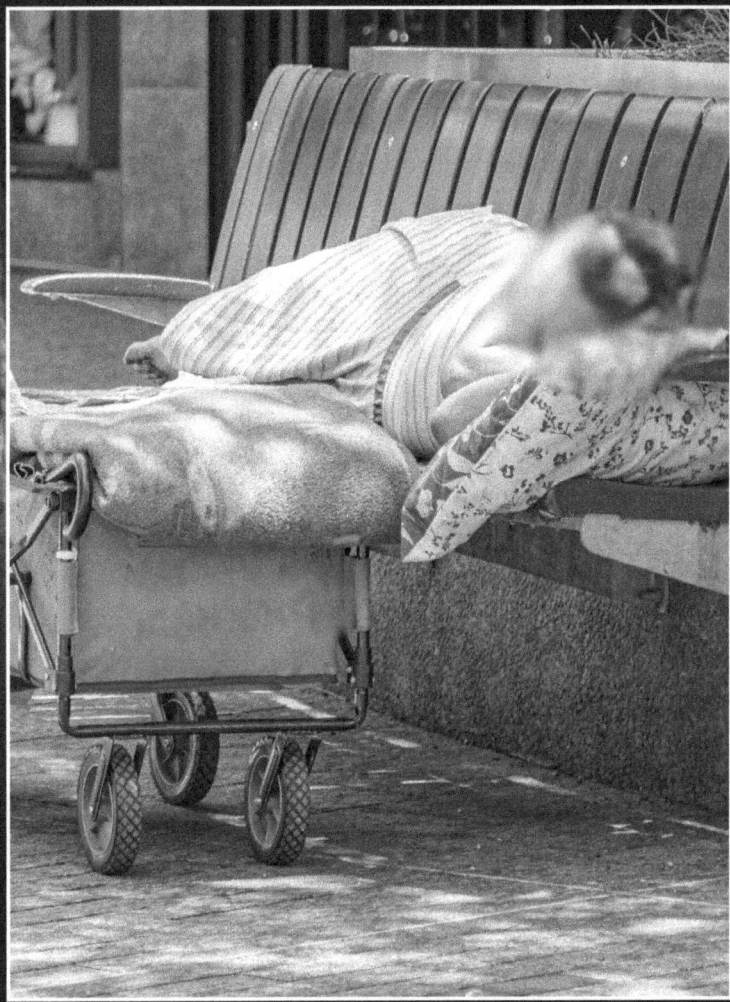

CHAPTER 2

Is our health actually getting worse?

The answer to this is yes and no.

In my opinion, Queensland and Australia have some of the best health systems and services in the world. We have some of the most highly trained and skilled health professionals who work within a mostly fair system. In my experience, clinicians in this country are mostly well intended and want to do the right thing. In my 22 years of working in a hospital setting, I have never once come across a clinician, food service officer, cleaner, wards person, administration officer or other hospital worker, who didn't want to do the right thing by their patients. The way patients are treated, the evidence-based treatments and access to services and medicines are good. I am so grateful for this.

However, it is preventative health that you will see improve and grow in the next years. This is because it's necessary. Preventing diseases before they occur is in focus. There are several reasons for this.

Firstly, many chronic diseases are preventable, yet many are growing in numbers. Understanding the way in which we prevent unhealthy behaviours leading to disease, will be paramount to improving the health of the population.

Secondly, many diseases are inequitable. That is, the risk of chronic disease within certain population groups remains higher than others. Reasons for this are complicated and of course, strongly linked to the social determinants of health. However, I have tried to outline some of the top issues we should focus on (and have already started).

Again, COVID-19 has taught us a few lessons. Evidence points to some population groups having been disproportionately affected (either directly or indirectly) by the COVID-19 pandemic – making its impact one of inequality. The indirect impacts extend to the social determinants of health, which include adverse effects on income, education, employment, housing and social connections – and these effects can influence health for many years into the future. Many vulnerable groups have been at a substantially increased risk during the pandemic, including Aboriginal and Torres Strait Islander people, people living with a disability and people with pre-existing health conditions – the communities that I worry about.

1. **Increased reports of poor mental health**.
    It would come as no surprise to you that COVID-19 appears to have impacted our mental health negatively. There were many reasons for this including the fear of the virus itself, being fined for breaching lockdown boundaries, your contact tracing data being reported on the news, from the stories from overseas of doctors choosing who was to be ventilated and who wasn't. It was truly the fear of the unknown.

Then came the debate about the vaccines. Which vaccine, the safety of the vaccines, news stories being shared of Australians allegedly dying of heart failure or allergic reactions to the vaccines, and then the desperate viewing of the daily numbers and the hope they would go down. The newfound popularity of the 'armchair epidemiologists' and their uninformed opinions being shared in workforces, pilates studios and children's schools continued to increase. Fear of the unknown affected all of us in such different ways. Fake news ran rife.

Lastly, the way the media called all of us to watch for the numbers, the stories and the devastation every day, didn't help.

As it was, our mental health was already fragile. In 2017-18, "23 per cent of Queensland adults reported a long-term mental health or behavioural problem, a prevalence that has more than doubled since 2001"[13] and this was prior to the pandemic.

One-in-13 (8%) 11–17-year-olds had a major depressive disorder, with the prevalence higher in girls aged 16-17 years (20%).[13] According to the ABS 2017–18 National Health Survey, more than one-quarter (26%) of Australians aged 15–24 (males 21%, females 30%) were experiencing a mental health or behavioural condition.[14] More than two-in-five (43.7%) Australians aged 16–85 had struggled with their mental health during their lifetime.[15]

That was all prior to COVID.

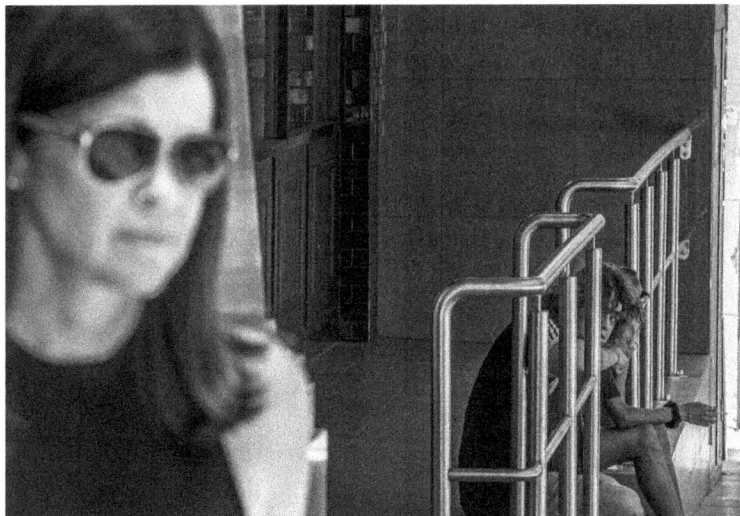

"A survey of Australians aged 15–19 years conducted between April and August 2020 found that more than two-in-five (43%) reported that they felt stressed, either all the time or most of the time, while a repeat study in 2021 found that 45 per cent rated their mental health as poor".[14]

The proportion of the adult population experiencing severe psychological distress was higher in April 2022 (11.6%) than it was prior to the pandemic (8.4% in February 2017) [16] and this continued to rise throughout the entire period.

"The reasons for the trend of increasing psychological distress among Australia's young people are unclear, but likely to be complex and vary between individuals".[14] A major finding out of this period was the psychological impacts on young people.

A study of 760 Australians aged 12–18 found that three-quarters (75%) felt that the COVID-19 pandemic had negatively impacted their mental health.[14] Our young people were and still are clearly at risk. This keeps me up at night.

The knowledge that our population is worried about their own wellbeing, yet many not being 'able' to do something about it, confirms my argument of the perfect storm. We are so vulnerable and dependent on the factors making up where we live. Our environment exerts such great forces on us and often completely removes our choices albeit through location, cost, weather or access. COVID-19 created power behind those forces. Life was busy and hard previously. We were all feeling a little vulnerable prior to 2019. I know I was. The pandemic came at a time where this cumulative impact could have maximum impact. This is exactly what happened.

I think there is much more to understand about why suicide in Queensland and Australia is high. Results revealing the COVID-19 pandemic impact are yet to be better understood. However, with nearly 800 Queenslanders taking their own lives every year, this remains unacceptable and so terribly tragic. It also leads me to believe that people are feeling out of control within their environment and their lives. I want this to change by creating the entire support we all need.

2. **Physical health is impacted by increased overweight and obesity rates** - in 2017-18, 65.9 per cent of Queensland adults aged older than 18 years were overweight (33.5%) or obese

(32.4%).[17] Among Queensland children aged 2-17 years, 24.5 per cent were overweight (15.4%) or obese (8.7%), in 2017-18.[17]

Research from My Health for Life conducted in April 2021, showed "almost half of Queenslanders surveyed reported to have gained weight, and 21 per cent reported a gain of more than five kilograms".[18]

Looking at more recent data for our state following the pandemic, the National Health Survey (NHS) revealed 69 per cent of the Queensland population was overweight (34%) or obese (35%) in 2022.[19]

No country or state has been able to reverse obesity rates in the long-term. In fact, at an individual, family, community, state, national and international level, reversing obesity has been unattainable.

Obesity is an intractable problem for our health system, for our economic wellbeing and for us. It is a pandemic in itself, which doesn't appear to have the urgency, the transparency and the reality that pandemics have received.

Obesity hurts. It impacts every single part of our body, our community, and our environment. It is the barrier to being able to live a healthy life, a longer life and an even happier life. According to Tam et al (2020), it has been shown that obesity reduces life expectancy by 5.8 years in men and 7.1 years in women after the age of 40.[20] Shorter life expectancy could be because obesity holistically accelerates ageing at multiple levels.[20] Besides jeopardising nuclear DNA and mitochondrial DNA integrity, obesity modifies the DNA methylation pattern, which is associated with epigenetic ageing in different tissues.[20] In simpler terms, obesity affects our DNA and so has a consequent impact on various aspects of the ageing process.

The causes of increased rates of overweight and obesity in any society are complex and nobody individually is to blame for the change. People are simply following the marketing messages which are often misleading and inaccurate. In fact, I don't know how anyone is still able to maintain a healthy weight.

3. **Increased diabetes rates** - The prevalence of diabetes in Queensland has increased by 58 per cent from 2001 to 2018-19.[13] Since 2001, this rate has increased from 3.3 per cent, however, has remained relatively stable since 2014-15 (5.1%).[21] One-in-20 (5.3%) people had diabetes in 2020-21 in Australia.[22] The detailed figures show that men are more likely to have diabetes than women and the risk increases with age.

No other single disease condition shares the same incredibly high rates of disease within the population. The sheer impact on most parts of the body including physical and mental health and the significant cost and demand to the health system is extraordinary. Many of us share the personal crises associated with living with the disease, or supporting family members who require treatment and support in one way or another. However, there is hope. Numerous large-scale randomised trials in many countries have shown that progression to type 2 diabetes may be delayed or prevented in up to 58 per cent of people with impaired glucose tolerance (pre-diabetes).[23] Diabetes is clearly an outcome of the environment that we live. Nobody wants diabetes. Nobody asks to endure the limitations and suffering it inflicts. Yet it is inequitably distributed and highly preventable. This is where we need to keep our focus. It is fixable if we know the data including the causes, the rates and the impacts of our environment.

WHAT THIS MEANS FOR YOUR VILLAGE:
The diseases that are most common in our country are preventable. Understanding the environment, the things that make it harder to be healthier (to eat well, to move a little more and to seek support and access to health services), ensures you not only know what you're dealing with, but also how to deal with it. This is empowerment at its best and I believe it's what's missing from our world right now.

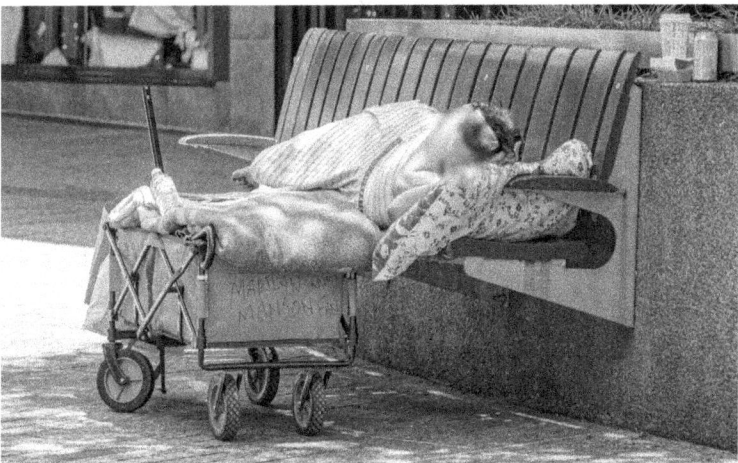

Chapter 2 References

13. Queensland Health. 2020. Report of the Chief Health Officer Queensland, the health of Queenslanders 2020.

14. Australian Institute of Health and Welfare. 2022. *Australia's health 2022, data insights: Mental health of young Australians* [Online]. Available: https://www.aihw.gov.au/getmedia/ ba6da461-a046-44ac-9a7f-29d08a2bea9f/aihw-aus-240_ Chapter_8.pdf.aspx [Accessed 8].

15. Australian Institute of Health and Welfare. 2022. *Mental health: prevalence and impact* [Online]. Australian Government. Available: https://www.aihw.gov.au/reports/mental-health-services/mental-health [Accessed 2023].

16. Australian Institute of Health and Welfare. 2022. *Australia's Health 2022: in brief* [Online]. Available: https://www.aihw. gov.au/getmedia/c6c5dda9-4020-43b0-8ed6-a567cd660eaa/ aihw-aus-241.pdf.aspx?inline=true [Accessed Australia's health series number 18].

17. Australian Bureau of Statistics. 2017-18. *Health conditions and risks - Overweight and obesity* [Online]. ABS. Available: https://www.abs.gov.au/statistics/health/health-conditions-and-risks/overweight-and-obesity/latest-release#cite-window2 [Accessed 2023].

18. Health and Wellbeing Queensland. 2021. *Obesity and COVID-19: It's time to double down* [Online]. Available: https:// hw.qld.gov.au/blog/obesity-and-covid-19-its-time-to-double-down/ [Accessed 2023].

19. Australian Bureau of Statistics. 2022. *National Health Survey, Summary Health Characteristics, States and Territories* [online]. Available: https://www.abs.gov.au/statistics/health/health-conditions-and-risks/national-health-survey/latest-release#data-downloads [Accessed 2024].

20. Tam, B. T., Morais, J. A. & Santosa, S. 2020. Obesity and ageing: Two sides of the same coin. *Obesity Reviews,* 21, e12991.

21. Australian Bureau of Statistics. 2017-18. *Diabetes* [Online]. ABS. Available: https://www.abs.gov.au/statistics/health/health-conditions-and-risks/diabetes/2017-18#cite-window1 [Accessed 2023].

22. Australian Bureau of Statistics. 2020-21. *Diabetes* [Online]. ABS. Available: https://www.abs.gov.au/statistics/health/health-conditions-and-risks/diabetes/latest-release [Accessed 2023].

23. Australian Government. 2021. *Australian National Diabetes Strategy* [Online]. Available: https://www.health.gov.au/sites/default/files/documents/2021/11/australian-national-diabetes-strategy-2021-2030_0.pdf [Accessed 2023].

CHAPTER 3

Fact vs Fiction. Creating solid
foundations for your village

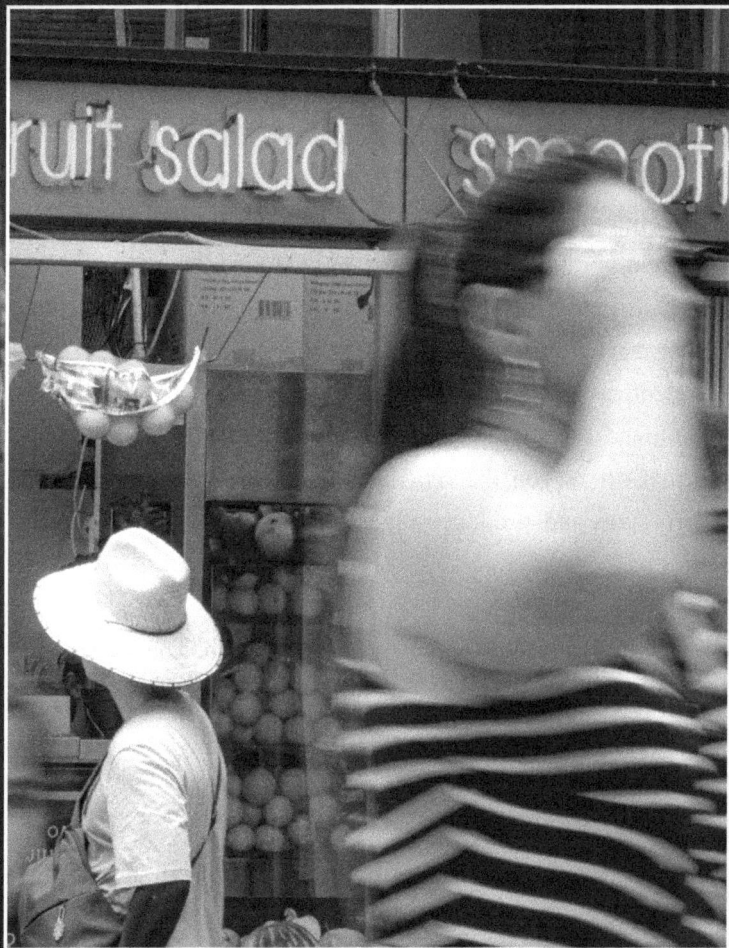

CHAPTER 3

Fact vs Fiction. Creating solid
foundations for your village

If there is one thing that bothers me more than the sheer volume of inaccurate information about nutrition out there, it's the deliberate intentions in which these myths are created.

The marketing giants of the current food industry are brilliant at their job. So good that even we, as trained professionals, find it incredibly difficult to sort fact from fiction. What's more, with the rapid pace that new products are added to our supermarkets, as well as the relentless reminders to buy and eat, it is almost impossible to recommend a completely updated, single 'go-to' information source that offers you the *real* information as the mountain of misinformation and product range for many commercial foods continues to grow.

Years ago, it was easier to spot a fad or a myth. Diets such as the 'cotton wool diet' and 'baby food diet' were easy to spot. They were as incorrect as they were overtly ridiculous and often completely unsafe.

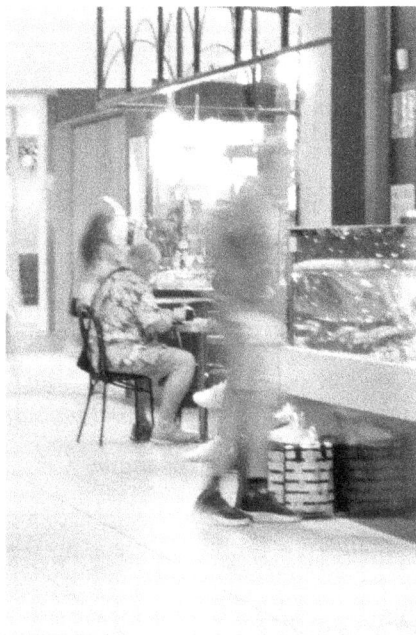

Today's marketing is quite brilliant in the most unfortunate way. Even some quite unsafe diets or approaches to dieting/ eating/exercising are seen to be underpinned by data and science. However, it's only when you look closely, that you understand this is not the case. Couple this with the cumulative effect of enormous marketing budgets of the fast-food industry and other unhealthy food companies (lollies, chocolates, soft drinks) and it is almost impossible to provide a defence.

This poses a major risk for health departments all around the world as they continue to fight against the incorrect messaging, the massive food industry budgets and the inequity of how this impacts on the health of our communities.

A. The volume of misinformation.

I once heard that in America, every 50 metres offers you a food cue. What that means is that on average, wherever you travel within the United States, there is a physical or digital sign reminding you to eat. Whether accurate or not, the sheer volume of advertising of food has become overwhelming. I do not know if the extent of the problem is the same for Australia or Queensland, but I am guessing we are not too far behind.

B. The food and fitness industry marketing budgets are enormous.

In the food industry, it is expected that the average company spends between three and six per cent of its overall revenue on marketing. However, some of the more well-known companies increase this to 10 per cent. For example, Coca-Cola spent $193 million U.S. in 2021 on advertising its priority beverage, while PepsiCo spent $114 million advertising the rival, Pepsi.[24]

Less than five years ago, it was reported in the Daily Mail, UK, that the advertising budget of 'junk food companies' was 27 times more than the amount the government used to promote healthy eating and there is proof of this occurring today.[25] More recently, in 2019, fast-food restaurants spent $5 billion in total advertising, an increase of more than $400 million (9%) vs. 2012.

C. Targeting of unhealthy products to vulnerable communities as priority

This is something I had to research to truly believe and the more I read, the more I was horrified. In America, a new study published by the University of Connecticut found that US food companies disproportionately marketed unhealthy food and drink, including candy, sodas, snacks and fast-food, to Black and Hispanic children, teens and adults.[27] Surely, that can't be the case in Australia... or so I hoped. In a scientific study by Brown in 2018, it was reported that there is a 'socioeconomic gradient' in TV viewing patterns for Australian children.[28] In other words, children from more vulnerable communities are more likely to watch TV and for longer periods of time, compared to their counterparts in more affluent areas. The most vulnerable children have a much greater exposure and thus, impact on their consumption of excessive fat, salt and sugar, from watching television with advertising. This drives the development of unhealthy, poor habits resulting in long-term health outcomes, often by stealth. This is exactly how inequity succeeds. These are the patterns that industry are well aware of as they collect data to show the trends.

Knowing these facts about children's viewing encourages some industry groups to take full advantage of such inequities. I am loath to share that a study (Settle et al, 2014), upon investigating outdoor food advertising found that at Melbourne transit stops, food advertisements are high.[29] This is not unexpected. However, 30 per cent of stops displayed food, with those in more disadvantaged suburbs more frequently promoting chain-brand fast food and less frequently promoting diet varieties of soft drinks.[29] Again, this is another example of inequity working against us – and our children. I hope this has both surprised you and motivated you to the point that you actively do something about it. It certainly has that effect on me. You need to stop blaming yourself for picking up fast foods on the way home as it is exactly what you're being told to do, how to do it and how you can pay for it!

The health food industry, the weight loss industry and the fitness industry are thriving, yet our incidence of preventative chronic diseases such as diabetes is increasing. What does that tell us? It's clear, it's not working for us. It's working against us.

It's time to understand the real facts.

Throughout my practice, the top 10 things people have misunderstood are listed below. I hope you find it helpful that I bust these myths for you. Again, please don't feel bad if you didn't have these right. Marketing, commercials and misinformed 'experts' may have just planned for you to get this wrong, so, basically, you were believing what you've been told!

1. **Muscle weighs more than fat - true**
    "Skeletal muscle is the largest organ in the human body accounting for about 40–50% of total weight in physiological conditions".[30] However, you don't want to lose skeletal muscle regardless of what it weighs as it is the organ that increases your metabolic rate (i.e. the higher the skeletal muscle, the higher your metabolic rate will be). In other words, the more skeletal muscle you have, the more effectively your body will burn energy. "Skeletal muscle is also essential for mobility and plays a major role in glycaemic control accounting for

up to 75 per cent of tissue glucose uptake".[31] Physical activity and training can increase your skeletal muscle mass and this is why physical activity is so important, especially as you age.[31] "Together, the two organs, the skeletal muscle and the heart, account for almost 30 per cent of resting energy consumption and nearly 100 per cent of increased energy consumption during exercise".[32]

Basically, it weighs more and the higher the skeletal muscle mass your body has, the more efficient your body is.

2. **I should do Keto – the jury is out......**
    The ketogenic diet is one of reduced carbohydrates and higher fat, but lower in calories, which leads to a state of ketosis.[33] The classic ketogenic diet (cKD) has been used to treat epilepsy in children continuously since 1921. My team and I have used this diet throughout our clinical services in hospitals successfully treating children with epilepsy, but only under the management of the medical and dietetic team.[33]

However, it is a very difficult to find clear rationale and reasoning to recommend this diet in the short-term and the long-term. I want to explain this.

The ketogenic diet has been shown to influence weight and conditions, such as obesity, insulin resistance and dyslipidaemia.[33] Interestingly, in many research reports, it is the effect on the gut (microbiota) that is reported as the actual factor that causes such beneficial changes in our body; not the diet itself.[33]

In many studies, there is a clear requirement for more research to be progressed to understand the true effect of the diet, its key characteristics (i.e. lower carbohydrate, higher protein and fat) and the effect on the metabolism, including the gut microbiota.[33] A recent study from Spain reported that a very low-calorie ketogenic diet (over four months) did in fact cause rapid weight loss, but also significantly changed the gut flora (microbiota) in terms of increasing diversity found in the gut.[33] What this means long-term is still not exactly clear.

After working at a children's hospital for so long, I was surprised to see such interest in the ketogenic diet by people who wanted to lose weight. I am often asked about its effectiveness (will it make me lose weight?), however, I am rarely asked about its safety. This is where I believe we need to be careful.

Firstly, in my opinion, the ketogenic diet works because it gives you fewer calories per day. Ultimately, reduced calories will cause weight loss, regardless of the way you do it, i.e. energy in = energy out.[34]

However, I believe the question should be - does the new composition of the diet (less carbohydrate and higher fat) produce some kind of scientific, chemical or metabolic effect that makes it even more efficient for weight loss, when compared to a regular low-calorie diet? I am yet to be convinced of this. In other words, is there a magical combination within the ketogenic diet that makes it more effective or is it simply the fact the diet provides fewer calories?

Another alternative view is that there is increased success of using this diet which is linked to the higher fat and protein consumption causes increased satiety (i.e., you feel full for longer).[33] However, I am very concerned about the long-term potential impact of this diet. I would question both the high protein load on the body and its potential effect on our kidney function and also the low fibre content. What does that do to our protective effects for cancer within our gut/digestive system? I have always lived by the quote "if you look after your gut, your gut will look after you". I don't know who said that, but I have heard that many times throughout my training. It has been a basic principle of my work since I can remember, and I think it is safe and effective. I have shared this with so many of my patients throughout the years.

Overall, with regard to this diet, the research is contradictory at best. One study proposes that "a ketogenic diet has the potential to alter the gut microbiota composition and function, thereby promoting alpha diversity but also the production of beneficial microbial metabolites".[33] In direct contrast, another study reports "that upon studying 91 Australian overweight or obese adults showed that an 8-week low-calorie and low-carbohydrate diet resulted in impaired bowel health, compared to an isocaloric high-carbohydrate diet".[33]

So one study is saying, by following a ketogenic diet, our gut health is improved, yet the other is saying our gut health is impaired. Trust me, the research here is not conclusive. If you are confused about the true effects of the ketogenic diet on weight, you are not alone.

If there is one thing that is clear, it is that short-, medium- and long-term studies are needed to understand both the benefits and the long-term impacts the ketogenic diet has on the body (if any).[33] It is the unknown nature and conflicting recommendations regarding the long-term use of this diet, that causes angst for me in recommending it. I would always try something different like this under full medical supervision - if you have to try it at all.

To be clear, the ketogenic diet supports weight loss. However, I believe, it is because of the reduction in calories, not the science within the diet itself that is the cause. If there is a lack of fibre in any diet, this is a red flag to me and as a result, I have never recommended to follow the ketogenic diet for weight loss personally.

3. **I should starve myself – false**
    The idea of starving has changed from when I first started working clinically as a dietitian. In the 1990s, I found so many cases where young people would try to starve themselves in the mornings by avoiding breakfast, only to find concentration at school and work was so affected that a larger, higher fat meal was consumed midmorning to counteract this. I will stand by what I said then. Starving is never the answer to long-term health. However, some forms of intermittent fasting, in my opinion, can be beneficial and safe (under close management). These are two very different things.

    Some examples of popular intermittent fasting include the alternate-day fasting, the 5:2 diet and time-restricted feeding - all of which produce mild to moderate weight loss (1-8%) as it also causes a reduction in energy intake (10-30%).

Remember, energy in = energy out.[34] Some scientific studies report metabolic benefits of intermittent fasting including a reduction in appetite and improved gut microbiome, as well as reduced blood pressure, insulin resistance and oxidative stress.[34] Low-density lipoprotein cholesterol and triglyceride levels have also been shown to reduce (aka good for your heart health). However, as variable as these diets are, so are the reported benefits.[34]

Generally, it is not something that I would recommend as critical to maintain a healthy body weight. I would continue to focus my energy on understanding marketing claims, reading labels and training myself to make very informed decisions on food preparation and choices, in the first instance. I feel this can never fail in the long-term and the extent of the problem and the impact is more far reaching than any other concern in our current diets.

4. **There are no superfoods – true. However, there are terrific foods to include in your diet for different reasons.**
    A superfood is a marketing term, often referring to the superior powers of a particular nutrient that is good for health and wellbeing. Most health professionals and dietitians do not refer to foods as superfoods. It is certainly not a term that I have ever used routinely, nor do I think there is a good, shared understanding or definition of what a superfood is. Be aware of the term and always read the labels. One thing is clear – 'superfoods' are highly variable in their superpowers. I am not saying these are not good foods but rather, take the time to understand why they are labelled a superfood and make an informed decision from there.

A word of caution; just because a food is labelled a superfood, it does not mean you can eat as much as you like. Often, because of the numerous benefits associated with the product, it is very concentrated or calorie dense as it contains such high-quality nutrition. This often comes with a very high calorie load. Please check you are not eating too much because you think it's healthy. I have fallen into that trap personally many times.

According to a recent study investigating the judgements of implied health terms, one common concern is that nutrition and health claims create the 'magic bullet' or 'halo' effects that lead consumers to believe that a food carrying such a claim is healthier than it actually is.[35] Variety is always best. In my opinion, there is no magic bullet or single food. Read labels carefully, especially those claiming health benefits.

If someone asked me if there was one superfood I ate regularly, I would also reply 'oats'. It is low in fat, high in fibre, good for balancing internal fats, versatile and fills you up. There are not many foods that do all of that.

5. **Coconut or banana bread, muffins and yoghurts are always healthy**
    If you are not gasping after you read the next few facts, then you are a better human than I! I am sure dietitians are not even as aware of these as they should be, simply because there are so many products coming to market every week. When you read below, please keep in mind adults require between 1,600-

3,000 calories per day, dependent on sex, age and physical activity levels.[36]

The caloric density of a slice of commercial coconut bread is: 680 calories[37,38,39,40,41]

The average caloric density of banana bread (retail) is: 470 calories.

The average caloric density of a 250g tub Greek yoghurt is: 300 calories[43,44,45,46,47]

The average caloric density of a commercial muffin is: 680 calories.

These figures mean that one commercial muffin or slice of coconut bread provides between 25 and 40 per cent of your total calorie needs for the entire day.

Labelling with words like gluten-free, fruit-based, and vegan-friendly are often added for unexpected reason, albeit, it is not incorrect. For example, I have seen an avocado in the past with a sticker on it which reads "this one has no saturated fat". Well, no avocados have saturated fat. However, this is a powerful marketing message and tool. I'm not saying that the marketing in this case was trying to be deceitful and I agree that avocados are good food. However, I am confident some companies do this intentionally to encourage us to buy more. Equally, lovely pictures of palm trees and farms are often provided on food labels for the same purpose. It is often to trick us into thinking they are entirely healthy, hoping you will buy more. Although, of course, this is not the case for all claims and labels. It is so difficult to understand which are accurate. Read food labels carefully and often make home-made products when you can. It is the only way you can be assured of the composition of the products. And yes, eat avocados. Although they contain about 20 per cent fat, it is a good fat that is good for your body. Using this as an alternative to saturated fats when you can is brilliant.

6. All salads are healthy – false

Working in a hospital and managing a café, I used to watch what everyone bought for lunch. What was clear to me, was that the majority of people wanted to be healthy. They were making conscious choices of what they believed to be healthy snacks and lunch products, such as caesar salads, salads with oil-based dressings and salads with a range of high-calorie/high-fat foods all mixed together. My colleagues worked really hard, were hungry and were often not entitled to another break until later that night. So, they bought what was available, what the marketing was telling them was good for them and continued to purchase the upsize or the drink combo (and another cappuccino on the side). A cappuccino wouldn't hurt when they were having salads for lunch…surely.

As the manager of the retail café, I introduced the old-fashioned but much-loved concept of the sandwich bar. This was where you would choose your bread and salads. As the chief dietitian, I used to love spending time in the café, especially during the lunch shift so I could provide caloric advice as I was serving customers. The introduction of the salad bar and other true health offerings supported the café to triple the profits it was making previously. I couldn't believe it. My learnings from this time:

1. We all tend to find comfort in the marketing supporting us to buy products they claim as 'healthy', even when we may not be 100 per cent sure it is. If you look hard enough, you can probably find a claim that will confirm inaccurate information.
2. Commercially prepared salads can have quadruple the calories, fat and also the nutrition, including energy, compared with others. Salads vary greatly.
3. People actually enjoy low-fat, freshly prepared, high-fibre options when they had a choice i.e. when they were fast and affordable.

Again, people want to be healthy and will choose healthy when it's easy. I strongly believe people would choose healthy options if they were just as fast, affordable, and convenient as take-aways. I have seen this throughout my career. However, I think we need to do better to ensure we offer this to everyone.

What I like about salads is the variety they bring. My top tips to salads are to ensure lots of colours, seasonal, lots of fibre-containing fresh or frozen foods and try to make your salads in house so you have control on what goes in.

The following examples may also surprise you, but they are completely true. These are examples of salads I have bought commercially from a very well-known Australian retailer:
The caloric density of a grilled chicken salad (retail) is: 470 calories.

The caloric density of a chicken, bacon and avocado salad (retail) is: 840 calories.

The caloric density of a chickpea salad (retail) is: 480 calories.

Below is a simple little calculation allowing you to see how salads' caloric density can vary significantly, especially when you compare homemade ingredients to commercial bought salads. Further, store bought salads are often expensive. It is the one item I don't remember ever buying already prepared. The cost, the nutrients, the additives, and the convenience, just don't add up to me when considering catering either for my family or parties. The pleasure and enjoyment of seeing a salad come together with layers, colours, textures, and tastes is brilliant. It seems almost disappointing when transferring a store-bought salad from a plastic container to a serving dish. In looking at the comparison, every commercial salad provided more than double the caloric density of the home made fresh salad.

Calculations:

Standard Homemade Salad	
2 cups leafy greens	14 calories
5 cherry tomatoes	2 calories
1 small chicken breast	160 calories
1/3 cup brown rice	92 calories
2 tbs balsamic vinegar	20 calories
Total	*290 calories*

224% more calories in the average restaurant/takeaway salad

Restaurant Caesar Salad	
Example 1	707 calories
Example 2	622 calories
Example 3	629 calories
Average	*650 calories*
Standard ingredients: Crumbed chicken, bacon, egg, parmesan, croutons, creamy dressing, lettuce	

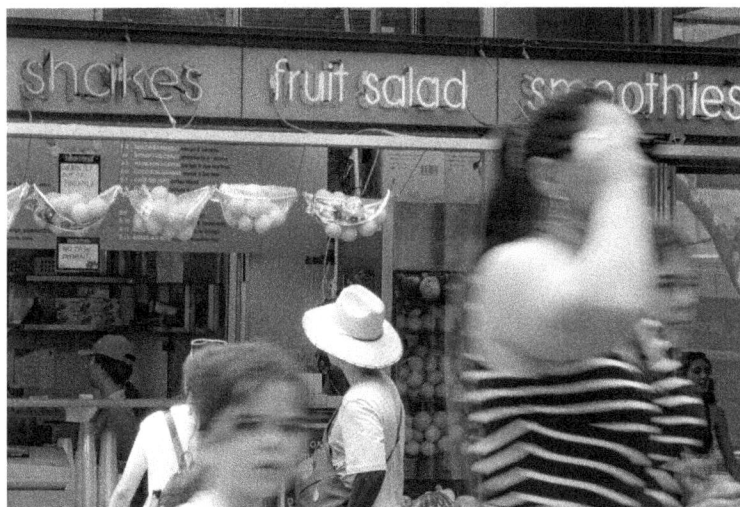

7. Juice is the same as fruit - false

As my children grew up, if they asked for a small amount of orange juice occasionally, I would give it to them but only a very small amount mixed with water. I never realised this was how they perceived that juice occurred naturally. When out for a buffet breakfast, my then 7-year-old son asked me why the orange juice tasted so thick as it was the first time he had tried full strength juice. I told him, it was because they added a lot of additional sugar to it. I wasn't wrong.

Juice is fruit minus the fibre. The sugar in fruit juice is often naturally occurring. However, that does not mean it is entirely good for you. In fact, several scientific studies have shown that fruit juice consumed daily may increase your blood pressure, with one study reporting an increase of 3–4 mmHg higher for those who consumed fruit juice daily, rather than rarely or occasionally.[49] It is well known that high sugar intake raises insulin levels. It has been proposed that this can lead to an increase in blood pressure and heart rate.

Did you know that it takes around three oranges to make only one cup of orange juice? We all know there is a considerable amount of naturally occurring sugar called fructose in oranges. How much do you think is in three?

Well, the answer is 14g sugar in 250mls of pure orange juice, which is three-and-a-half teaspoons. Adding to this, a serve of orange juice sold commercially is usually a lot larger than 250mls.

In my opinion, fruit juice is one of those products that I do not see value for our children or the entire population overall. It is an easy way to consume high volumes of sugar (natural or added) and has been the subject of a great number of marketing campaigns urging you to drink more. If you are eating fruit, juice is simply not needed.

8. Standing desks are a good idea – true
I very much endorse!

I stand all day at work. I first heard of a standing desk about five years ago. I tried it for a day, my legs ached, and I thought

I would never try it again. Today, I don't even have a chair in my office. I have a high stool for when I want to take a longer meeting, but I refuse to sit for long periods ever during the day. Long-term standing helps me with my posture, my energy levels and my ability to pivot across the office to different events as I need to. More importantly, I am stronger and clearer in my discussions when I am standing. Standing symmetrically and structurally supports diaphragmatic breath (not chest breath), assisting in voice projection and clarity of speech. This simple change in my life has helped me with both my physical and mental health. It sounds ridiculous, but I am such a convert and can never go back.

Here are some facts about standing desks.

Sitting requires less energy. When standing, there are two things that are occurring. You are using approximately 21 per cent more energy (that can vary in the literature) and you are also using (contracting and activating) muscles in your body you wouldn't otherwise use when sitting.

Our world has become much more reliant on sitting and passive work. The more we can change the environment to allow us to move, stand, walk and improve our overall balance and posture, the better.

I use a standing desk at work every day. In fact, I don't convert my standing desk ever to a sit desk. I arrive in the morning in the office to a standing desk and I leave it in the same position. My screens are positioned for standing for meetings and even for keyboard use.

I ensure my entire workforce has access to a standing desk, can organise walking meetings on a regular basis and also has one free hour each day to move around or get outside for a walk.

Whether you work at home, in an office, in a ward or at a salon, the ability to stand for longer, move and stretch, is so critical to our long-term posture, good health and overall wellbeing. Some important quotes from the literature include:

- Excessive sitting time has been linked to an increased likelihood of many negative health outcomes, including mortality.[50]

- Those who sit from eight to 11 hours per day have an increased mortality rate by 15 per cent in the three years following, compared to those who sit for less than four hours.[50]

- In addition, obesity, type 2 diabetes, cancer and cardiovascular disease are more prevalent in those who spend excessive time sitting.[50]

- Office workers typically spend more than half of their day sitting, making them an at-risk group for developing sitting-related conditions.[50]

A systematic review revealed "prolonged sitting can potentially cause low back pain due to lumbar flexion" (also known as slouching).[51] A standing position inhibits lumbar flexion.[51] Periods of time on a standing workstation have shown to be preventive against such injuries at work.[51] Interestingly, contrary to a treadmill workstation, the upright posture from standing workstations does not alter executive office tasks, such as typing and mouse pointing.[51] Moreover, standing workstations do not increase perceived exertion or reduce the efficiency of computer tasks.[51] Furthermore, studies suggest that globally, standing workstations do not alter cognitive performance tasks.[51]

The use of standing desks is being much more closely researched, as the benefits are starting to become clear. In the classroom, there have been reports of increased physical activity and energy expenditure, as well as better classroom behaviour in children using standing desks.[52] As a student (and I was studious, focused and hard-working), I found sitting still the hardest thing throughout the entirety of my study years. From Year 1 and throughout all of my university lectures, I found sitting, writing and concentrating, did not agree with me. My legs felt heavy, and I used to describe the feeling that "my legs wanted to go for a run on their own". I was always restless and as a result, I was often in trouble for not sitting still. I am still well known for fidgeting if I am sitting and that has never changed, so why not use it all to our advantage.

This is just another example of questioning what we do because we've always done it that way. What if kids stood at a desk, moved around the classroom more and had many more physical activity breaks? I feel the outcomes would speak for themselves.

9. Gluten free is much healthier – false

When I was training to become a dietitian, one of my assignments was to follow a very restricted diet. My diet assignment was to remain gluten-free for two weeks. This was probably the most difficult project I have ever completed. I loved (and still do) just about every form of carbohydrate. I enquired at a bakery if they had any gluten-free products, in which they advised "gluten is in the air and these products simply didn't exist". This is completely inaccurate and clearly specialised diets were not well known 25 years ago. I love carbohydrates and to change to an almost carbohydrate free diet overnight, was the most energy-reducing, depressing, and emotional-impacting change I have ever experienced. I have never forgotten it and learned several things during this experience:

1. Things have significantly improved for people requiring gluten-free diets in the past 25 years. Phew!

2. However, some people still don't understand exactly what gluten-free is. Read labels, check ingredients and home-bake to be sure when you can.

3. As a dietitian, doctor, carer, mother or friend, please don't recommend a gluten-free diet unless it is medically indicated or specifically helpful for the individual. Such a radical change can impact someone's physical and mental health. If necessary, such a significant restriction should be considered and planned carefully under medical advice.

4. To provide gluten-free products, many bakeries replace the carbohydrate with fat. Friands are a wonderful example of a tasty gluten-free, high-fat, moreish substitute for bread and/or cakes. Friands provide approximately 320 calories and 20g of fat, compared with a crumpet which provides about a quarter of the calories.

5. Following strict gluten free diets can support your body to gain weight. I did in one week.

Before we discuss gluten free products, let's discuss why people need to adhere to such a restrictive diet.

For those medically trained, it is accepted that coeliac disease is a "systemic immune-mediated disease caused by gluten and related prolamins in genetically susceptible individuals and is characterized by the presence of a variable combination of gluten-dependent clinical manifestations, enteropathy, specific antibodies and HLA–DQ2 or HLA–DQ8 haplotypes. Despite differences in pathological mechanisms, clinical manifestations, and epidemiology, the treatment of all gluten-related disorders (GRDs) consists of excluding gluten-containing cereals and by-products from the diet, which affects almost 10 per cent of the population".[53]

In other words, coeliac disease is a serious autoimmune disease where the ingestion of gluten found in wheat, rye and barley, causes the body to produce an immune response that attacks its own cells, causing damage to the villi (the finger like projections that line the small intestine and absorb nutrients). Coeliac disease is hereditary and those with a first-degree relative have a 10 per cent chance of developing the disease in their lifetime.

This is different from gluten intolerance.

Gluten intolerance is described as "an onset of a spectrum of clinical manifestations in response to the ingestion of wheat, rye and barley in the absence of coeliac disease and wheat allergy... which is characterised by sensitivity to gluten proteins found in wheat, barley and rye, in subjects who test negative for coeliac disease and wheat allergy, respectively".[54] An adherence to gluten-free diet on a lifelong basis is the only proven effective treatment for gluten intolerance and other wheat associated disorders, because it only takes small amounts of gluten to cause considerable problems.[54] I have never recommended a gluten-free diet to anyone other than for these reasons. However, as you would have seen in the supermarket, over the past few years, more and more gluten-free products have become available. It is concerning to me that there is public perception that a gluten-free diet provides health benefits, including weight loss.

Unfortunately, the increased availability of gluten-free products has not been able to keep up with the rigour required to ensure nutrition adequacy. In other words, the science behind the products hasn't kept up with the demand on our shelves. As a result, gluten-free products alone may not provide you with a nutrient balanced diet. "The results of several studies have revealed that nutritional deficiencies can be produced due to the consumption of gluten-free diets in terms of calories, vitamins, minerals, dietary fibre and protein".[54] The research is suggesting evidence of nutritional deficiencies. Of most concern, iron, calcium and magnesium deficiencies are evident.[54] Numerous authors claim that gluten-free diets are inadequate in folate, B complex vitamins and protein.

A 2013 nutrition survey including 58 healthy adults showed that men following a gluten-free diet consumed significantly lower amounts of carbohydrates, fibre, niacin, folate and calcium, but significantly higher amounts of fat and sodium, than men eating a gluten containing diet (GCD).[55] Women eating a gluten-free diet consumed significantly lower amounts of carbohydrates, fibre, folate, iron and calcium, but significantly more fat, saturated fat and cholesterol, than women eating a GCD.[55] Overall, adults adhering to a gluten-free diet did not consume enough nutrient-dense foods to meet all nutritional recommendations.[55]

Again, people are listening to what they believe is true. They have heard that gluten-free is best and provides us with health benefits, when in fact, it may be the opposite.

To be clear, for those requiring a gluten-free diet for clinical purposes, I feel the current offerings have progressed in leaps and bounds. The diet has much more range and diversity and commercial products are now of excellent quality and diversity. It is also assumed that people with gluten intolerance or coeliac disease are under the care of a medical officer.

For all others, I say buyer beware. However, none of this is your fault. If you are buying gluten-free products because you've heard it's better for you, you are simply doing what you've been told. It's who is telling you this information that needs consideration. Check the labels and the reasons why you chose to follow a gluten-free diet in the first place and this will empower you and your village to choose wisely into the future. Who will benefit?

10. Fats and oils are good for you – true and false.

We live in a world where incredibly clever food marketers are allowed to strategically use words like 'lite' or 'extra lite' to refer to colour rather than caloric density (which is exactly the point of the marketing). Again, this is another area where marketing is unethical and quite relentless in its targeting of people who are most vulnerable.

Rule number one. Fat is fat. It will cause weight gain if eaten in excess, regardless of the type. One gram of fat or oil provides you with nine calories or 37.7kjoules of energy. This is higher compared to one gram of carbohydrate or protein which provides four calories or 16.7kjoules per gram which is less than half that of fat. Basically, fat provides you more than double the amount of energy, compared to other foods of the same weight. However, this section is not talking about weight gain. I would like to explain the benefits of fats and oils in our diets. Just be aware, it will always have the same caloric density.

We, as dietitians, have a way of making things quite complicated. To be clear, it's never because we don't want to do the right thing. In fact, it's because we want to do the right thing always and give you so much more information than you probably need to know. This section is designed to make the information easier to understand but also easier for you to make decisions, as you work hard to prepare healthy food for your family.

To easily understand the impacts of fats and oils, you need to understand two things:

1. **The truth about your own body's fats and how our diet affects this.**
   Fats in the blood are called lipids. Lipids in your blood join with proteins which are then called lipoproteins (also known as cholesterol). There are four types in your blood:

   a. High density lipoproteins (HDL) – AKA 'good cholesterol'
   b. Low density lipoproteins (LDL) – AKA 'bad cholesterol'
   c. Very low-density lipoproteins (VLDL)
   d. Triglycerides (TG) – another type of fat in the blood, caused by habitual overeating[56]

There are two things you need to look for when understanding your cholesterol readings from your doctor:
   o The total cholesterol number is the reading you get from the doctor. Basically, the lower the better. The overall level should not exceed 5.5mmol/L.[57] Any number above this level is when you should be considering seeing your GP more often and where you will be guided to consider diet or medication treatment.

As a major health concern in Australia, approximately half of all Australian adults have a blood cholesterol level above 5mmol/L.[58]

o   The ratio of blood cholesterol is critical. The lower the LDL, VLDL and TG and the higher the HDL, is what you want to see. Basically, these are the levels you would want to aim for (as these indicate good healthy ratios):

    a.   HDL: >1.0mmol/L[57]
    b.   LDL: <2.0mmol/L[57]
    c.   VLDL: 0.1 – 1.7 mmol/L[59]
    d.   TG: <1.7mmol/L[56]

2. **The difference in fats and oils. This is often as simple as understanding the differences in the physical appearance of the fats and oils you buy.**
I will start this section by defining the different types of fats.

*   **Unsaturated fats** are the 'good fats'. These fats generally increase your HDL levels and decrease your LDL and VLDL.[60]

*   They are generally obtained from plants or fish and usually appear as liquid at room temperature. Examples include olive oil and the fats from avocados and nuts.[60]

    o   High concentrations of monounsaturated fats are found in olives, peanut and canola oils, avocados, almonds, hazelnuts and pecans, pumpkin and sesame seeds.[61]

    o   High concentrations of polyunsaturated fats are found in sunflower, corn, soybean and flaxseed oils, walnuts, flaxseeds, fish and canola oil.[61]

o   Omega-3 fats are an important type of polyunsaturated fat. We must obtain these types of fat from food as they can't be made by our body.[61] An excellent way to get omega-3 fats is by eating fish 2-3 times a week, or from plant sources including flax seeds, walnuts, and canola or soybean oil.[61] Higher blood omega-3 fats are associated with lower risk of premature death among older adults, according to a study by The Harvard School of Public Health.[61] "The omega−3 (n−3) polyunsaturated fatty acids (PUFAs) eicosapentaenoic acid (EPA) and docosahexaenoic acid (DHA) are well known to protect against numerous metabolic disorders".[62]

- **Saturated fats** are solid at room temperature. They increase your LDL and VLDL and decrease your HDL. This is exactly what you don't want. These are usually found in animal sources, coconut products and fats obtained from butter, cheese, some chocolate and products containing palm oil.[60]

- **Trans fats** (or trans fatty acids) are man-made and are banned in some countries. Hydrogen is forced into liquid vegetable oils, resulting in a more solid fat. According to the Harvard School of Public Health "they are the worst type of fat for the heart, blood vessels, and rest of the body because they raise bad LDL, create inflammation (a reaction related to immunity – which has been implicated in heart disease), stroke, diabetes, and other chronic conditions, contribute to insulin resistance and are harmful to health in even small amounts. So much so, for each additional two per cent of calories from trans fat consumed daily, the risk of coronary heart disease increases by 23 per cent".[61] Some common products that contain trans fats include fried foods, baked goods, processed snack foods and margarine.[61]

Some interesting facts on fat:

- Solid fats can start out as liquid fats and through a process called hydrogenation, they become more saturated than unsaturated.[61] Basically, their structure changes from a liquid to a solid at room temperature. A good example of this is when we use cooking oil in the kitchen (or at fish and chip restaurants). The first time we use it to fry food, the oil is a healthy one. The more we heat oil, the more it solidifies and more it becomes saturated – thus, an unhealthy fat.[61]

- Manufacturers are not required to declare trans fatty acids (TFAs) on the label, although they can provide this information voluntarily. In June 2015, the US Food and Drug Administration (US FDA) announced it had finalised its determination that partially hydrogenated oils (the primary source of manufactured TFAs) are no longer 'generally recognised as safe'.[63]

- While we are consuming levels of TFAs well below the WHO recommendation, we are still exceeding the recommendations in the Australian Dietary Guidelines and the New Zealand Food and Nutrition Guidelines, that saturated and TFAs combined contribute no more than 10 per cent of our daily energy intake.[64]

- According to many studies, the fatty acid profile and natural antioxidant content of extra virgin olive oil (EVOO) supports the oil to remain stable when heated, which continues to promote beneficial health outcomes. As a result, EVOO is a good oil to use and you should look for it specifically on restaurant menus now.

- There are 10 foods that can reduce bad cholesterol. However, the way they reduce cholesterol is variable. Out of all the foods listed below, oats are a wonderful food with many benefits due to their soluble fibre content. As I indicated in the previous section, if there was one item I would recommend adding to your diet every day, it would be natural oats. I eat them without fail on a daily basis.

1. Oats – due to the outstanding soluble fibre content.
2. Barley - again, they have a high soluble fibre content.
3. Beans - for the same reasons above - BUT there are so many other reasons here including protein and fibre.
4. Eggplant – great natural source of soluble fibre.
5. Nuts – the nutrients provide a protective effect. In fact, some very strong research in women showed that those who ate at least a quarter of a cup twice a week lowered their risk of death from cardiovascular disease by about one third.
6. Fruit – apples, grapes and strawberries are high in pectin, which is a type of soluble fibre.
7. Vegetable oils – olive oil, canola, sunflower and safflower oils added to salads will reduce your risk of cardiovascular disease.
8. Soy – soybeans and tofu.

9. Fatty fish – two or three times/week by increasing omega 3s.
10. Whole grains – such a wonderful source of soluble fibre.

What can we do for our village to prosper?

The learning here for me is that there are so many myths out there, I don't even correct people at BBQs anymore. My mother often looks at me and wonders why I don't simply say 'there is carbohydrate in bananas' and 'coconut water is not a superfood'. However, empowering you through some of these simple recommendations works better for me than anything else I can dispel in five minutes over a 'cauliflower rice salad'. Anyway, is it even a rice?

Most important tip here is to understand that marketing of unhealthy food such as fast-food marketing is a commercial determinant of health. This is a perfect example of how the food and beverage industry practices create conditions that drive consumption of highly processed foods and beverages. Be clear. They are deliberate in their strategies.

WHAT THIS MEANS FOR YOUR VILLAGE:
Question everything. Take the time to read the information, the data and privacy rules, the labelling and the expertise behind who is giving you the information and above all, question the motivation behind what you're experiencing. *Who is making money here?*

Chapter 3 References

24. Faria, J. 2023. *Ad spend of selected beverage brands in the US 2021* [Online]. Statista. Available: https://www.statista.com/statistics/264985/ad-spend-of-selected-beverage-brands-in-the-us/ [Accessed 2023].

25. Spencer, B. 2017. *Junk food companies' advertising budget is 27 TIMES bigger than cash the government uses to promote healthy eating* [Online]. Daily Mail Australia. Available: https://www.dailymail.co.uk/health/article-4968306/Junk-food-ads-spend-27-times-health-scheme.html [Accessed 2023].

26. Harris J, F.-M. F., Phaneuf L, Jensen M, Choi Y, Mccann M, Mancini S. 2021. *Fast Food Facts 2021. Fast food advertising: billions in spending, continue high exposure by youth.* [Online]. UConn Rudd Center for Food Policy & Obesity. Available: https://media.ruddcenter.uconn.edu/PDFs/FACTS2021.pdf [Accessed].

27. Rudd Center for Food Policy & Health. 2022. *Rudd Report Executive Summary – Targeted food and beverage advertising to black and Hispanic consumers: 2022 update.* [Online]. University of Connecticut. Available: https://uconnruddcenter.org/wp-content/uploads/sites/2909/2022/11/Rudd-Targeted-Marketing-Report-2022.pdf [Accessed 2023].

28. Brown, V., Ananthapavan, J., Veerman, L., Sacks, G., Lal, A., Peeters, A., Backholer, K. & Moodie, M. 2018. The Potential Cost-Effectiveness and Equity Impacts of Restricting Television Advertising of Unhealthy Food and Beverages to Australian Children. *Nutrients* [Online], 10.

29. Settle, P. J., Cameron, A. J. & Thornton, L. E. 2014. Socioeconomic differences in outdoor food advertising at public transit stops across Melbourne suburbs. *Australian and New Zealand Journal of Public Health,* 38, 414-418.

30. Biolo, G., Cederholm, T. & Muscaritoli, M. 2014. Muscle contractile and metabolic dysfunction is a common feature of sarcopenia of aging and chronic diseases: from sarcopenic obesity to cachexia. *Clinical nutrition (Edinburgh, Scotland),* 33, 737-748.

31. Mcgregor, R. A. & Poppitt, S. D. 2013. Milk protein for improved metabolic health: a review of the evidence. *Nutr Metab (Lond),* 10, 46.

32. Baskin, K. K., Winders, B. R. & Olson, E. N. 2015. Muscle as a "mediator" of systemic metabolism. *Cell Metab,* 21, 237-248.

33. Attaye, I., Van Oppenraaij, S., Warmbrunn, M. V. & Nieuwdorp, M. 2022. The Role of the Gut Microbiota on the Beneficial Effects of Ketogenic Diets. *Nutrients* [Online], 14.

34. Varady, K. A., Cienfuegos, S., Ezpeleta, M. & Gabel, K. 2021. Cardiometabolic Benefits of Intermittent Fasting. *Annual Review of Nutrition,* 41, 333-361.

35. Orquin, J. L. & Scholderer, J. 2015. Consumer judgments of explicit and implied health claims on foods: Misguided but not misled. *Food Policy,* 51, 144-157.

36. BUTLER, N. 2023. *How many calories should I eat a day?* [Online]. Medical News Today. Available: https://www. medicalnewstoday.com/articles/245588 [Accessed 2023].

37. Carb Manager. 2023. *Carbs in Liberated Coconut Bread* [Online]. Wombat Apps. Available: https://www.carbmanager.com/food-detail/ md:131d518b51a40fde7a6d08a25203ceb4/coconut- [Accessed 2023].

38. Nutritionix. 2023. *Coconut Bread - 1 piece* [Online]. A Syndigo Company. Available: https://www. nutritionix.com/i/nutritionix/coconut-bread-1- piece/5909e48a3a2b319e22f25df3 [Accessed 2023].

39. Fat Secret Australia 2023. *Coconut Bread Calories* [Online].

Available: https://www.fatsecret.com.au/calories-nutrition/
search?q=Coconut+Bread [Accessed 2023].

40. Eat This Much. 2023. *Coconut Bread* [Online]. Available:
https://www.eatthismuch.com/food/nutrition/coconut-
bread,2443539/ [Accessed 2023].

41. My Net Diary. 2023. *Toast'em Pandan Coconut Bread*
[Online]. Available: https://www.mynetdiary.com/food/
calories-in-toast-em-pandan-coconut-bread-by-gardenia-
slice-28396257-0.html [Accessed 2023].

42. Easy Diet Diary. 2023. Commercial Banana Bread (regular
Slice).

43. Burrell, S. 2022. *Your favourite muesli bars ranked by sugar,
from highest to lowest.* [Online]. Nine News. Available:
https://coach.nine.com.au/diet/muesli-bars-ranked-by-sugar-
australia-dietitian-susie-burrell/8b16d655-3e37-4e00-8632-
76513d985f5e [Accessed 2023].

44. Fat Secret Australia. 2023. *Uncle Toby's Muesli Bar*
[Online]. Fat Secret Australia. Available: https://www.
fatsecret.com.au/calories-nutrition/uncle-tobys/muesli-bar/1-
bar#:~:text=There%20are%20124%20calories%20in%20
1%20bar%20of%20Uncle%20Tobys%20Muesli%20Bar.
[Accessed 2023].

45. Calorie King. 2023. *Carman's Classic Fruit & Nut Muesli
Bar* [Online]. Calorie King. Available: https://www.
calorieking.com/au/en/foods/f/calories-in-bars-classic-fruit-
nut-muesli-bar/TVE11neTSP22Iqb_4GrGbQ [Accessed
2023].

46. Calcount. 2023. *Calories in Muesli Bar, Fruit & Nut*
[Online]. Calcount. Available: https://www.caloriecounter.
com.au/food/calories-in-muesli-bar-fruit-nut/ [Accessed
2023].

47. Eat This Much. 2023. *Muesli Bar - Oats and Seeds
Woolworths* [Online]. Eat This Much. Available: https://

www.eatthismuch.com/food/nutrition/muesli-bar,164039/ [Accessed 2023].

48. Easy Diet Diary. 2023. Easy Diet Diary. Commercial Berry Muffin (medium).

49. Pase, M. P., Grima, N., Cockerell, R. & Pipingas, A. 2015. Habitual intake of fruit juice predicts central blood pressure. *Appetite,* 84, 68-72.

50. Chambers, A. J., Robertson, M. M. & Baker, N. A. 2019. The effect of sit-stand desks on office worker behavioral and health outcomes: A scoping review. *Appl Ergon,* 78, 37-53.

51. Dupont, F., Léger, P. M., Begon, M., Lecot, F., Sénécal, S., Labonté-Lemoyne, E. & Mathieu, M. E. 2019. Health and productivity at work: which active workstation for which benefits: a systematic review. *Occup Environ Med,* 76, 281-294.

52. Minges, K. E., Chao, A. M., Irwin, M. L., Owen, N., Park, C., Whittemore, R. & Salmon, J. 2016. Classroom Standing Desks and Sedentary Behavior: A Systematic Review. *Pediatrics,* 137, e20153087.

53. Mármol-Soler, C., Matias, S., Miranda, J., Larretxi, I., Fernández-Gil, M. D. P., Bustamante, M., Churruca, I., Martínez, O. & Simón, E. 2022. Gluten-Free Products: Do We Need to Update Our Knowledge? *Foods,* 11.

54. Tanveer, M. & Ahmed, A. 2019. Non-Celiac Gluten Sensitivity: A Systematic Review. *J Coll Physicians Surg Pak,* 29, 51-57.

55. Kim, H. S., Demyen, M. F., Mathew, J., Kothari, N., Feurdean, M. & Ahlawat, S. K. 2017. Obesity, Metabolic Syndrome, and Cardiovascular Risk in Gluten-Free Followers Without Celiac Disease in the United States: Results from the National Health and Nutrition Examination Survey 2009-2014. *Dig Dis Sci,* 62, 2440-2448.

56. Victorian Government. 2021. *Triglycerides* [Online]. Better

Health Channel. Available: https://www.betterhealth.vic.gov. au/health/conditionsandtreatments/triglycerides [Accessed 2023].

57. Commonwealth Scientific Industrial Research. 2022. *Cholesterol Facts* [Online]. CSIRO. Available: https://www. csiro.au/en/research/health-medical/nutrition/cholesterol-facts#:~:text=Total%20Cholesterol%3A%20%3C4.0%20 mmol%2F,)%3A%20%3C%202.0%20mmol%2FL [Accessed 2023].

58. Victorian Government. 2021. *Cholesterol* [Online]. Better Health Channel. Available: https://www.betterhealth.vic.gov. au/health/conditionsandtreatments/cholesterol [Accessed 2023].

59. National Library of Medicine. 2023. *Cholesterol testing and results* [Online]. Available: https://medlineplus.gov/ency/ patientinstructions/000386.htm [Accessed 2023].

60. University of Minnesota. 2022. *What is the difference between fats and oils?* [Online]. Available: https:// reallifegoodfood.umn.edu/eat/nutrition/myplate/fats-and-oils [Accessed 2023].

61. Harvard University. 2023. *Types of Fat* [Online]. School of Public Health. Available: https://www.hsph.harvard.edu/ nutritionsource/what-should-you-eat/fats-and-cholesterol/ types-of-fat/ [Accessed 2023].

62. Saini, R. K., Prasad, P., Sreedhar, R. V., Akhilender Naidu, K., Shang, X. & Keum, Y.-S. 2021. Omega−3 Polyunsaturated Fatty Acids (PUFAs): Emerging Plant and Microbial Sources, Oxidative Stability, Bioavailability, and Health Benefits—A Review. *Antioxidants* [Online], 10.

63. European Commission. 2019. *Labelling Nutrition Trans Fats* [Online]. Available: https://food.ec.europa.eu/system/ files/2019-04/fs_labelling-nutrition_transfats_swd_ia-pt04. pdf [Accessed 2023].

64. Australian Institute of Health and Welfare. 2020. *Indicators for the Australian National Diabetes Strategy 2016–2020: data update* [Online]. Australian Government. Available: https://www.aihw.gov.au/reports/diabetes/diabetes-indicators-strategy-2016-2020/contents/goal-1-prevent-people-developing-type-2-diabetes/1-7-total-energy-intake-from-saturated-fatty-acids [Accessed 2023].

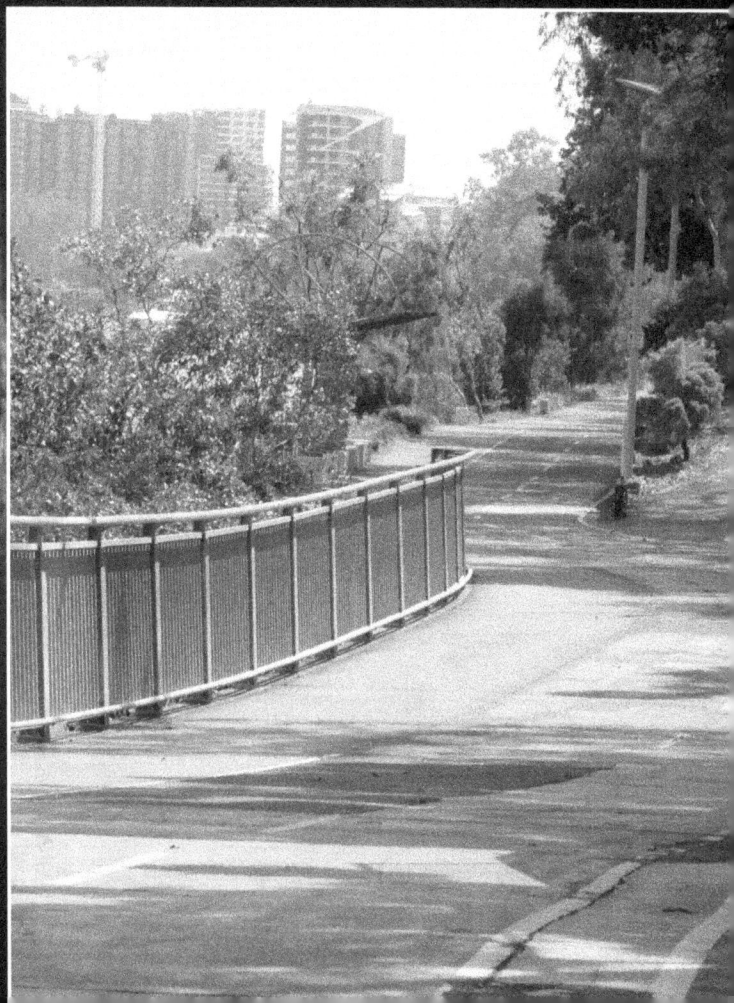

CHAPTER 4

Protecting your wellbeing

I go to Pilates nearly every day. I do that because it's indoors, it's warm and comfortable and I can work out at my own pace. Someone instructs me and supports everything I do for 40 minutes. I don't speak, there is no pressure on me to make decisions or sort through conflicts or respond to escalating issues. I am simply working hard physically, increasing my heart rate, enjoying a lovely, clean, nice-smelling environment, that offers soothing yet motivational music and lovely, encouraging instructors providing the best advice, catering to my individual needs and abilities through their dulcet tones, filling me with confidence and calm. Further, I leave the studio with a sense of empowerment as my body feels stronger, and more flexible, with an improvement in my fitness also emerging. I feel ready for the day and capable to work through whatever my life throws at me. My cup is full.

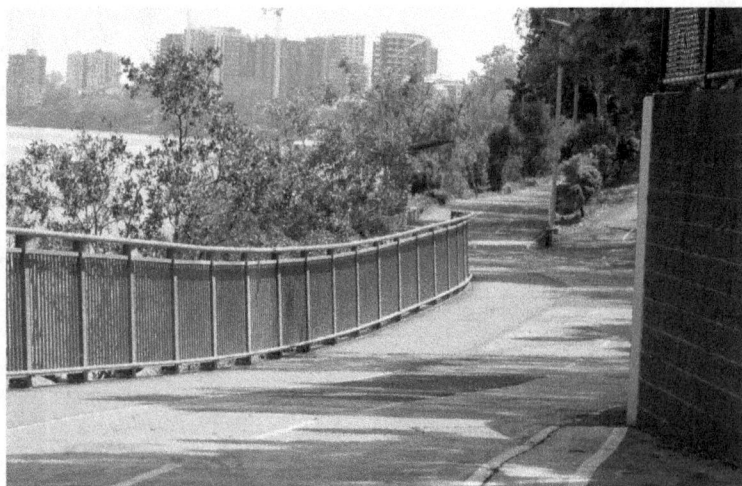

I run or walk three or four times per week. I find a gorgeous path, not too crowded, allowing me to enjoy my own pace. I can choose what I want to do, as my brain fires impulses to my body's tired and often sore muscles, advising whether to walk and relax or run at speed. Either way, this is never pre-determined before I start the activity. Some days I walk once around a 3km block and I feel good. I resist the temptation to continue to complete another few laps to reach the 10km mark because it's what's expected. Some days, I walk 20kms which takes me a few hours as I listen to music, someone reading me books or I talk to my dog as she pulls me in every direction. In any case, the only choice I make prior to going somewhere is that it must be peaceful, tree lined and if I get to the top of a hill, I will see a beautiful view. I call that 'my reward'.

This is how I view my exercise every day. I have found two activities that I love and have now become a part of my routine, my diary and my life. Everyone who knows me understands this comes first. This is completely my choice. This quarantined time in my day and the activities I am released to participate in every day ensures my wellbeing is good. In fact, this improves my health and wellbeing more than anything else in my whole life. If I can continue in this routine, I am a better mother, partner, daughter, friend and CEO. Yet, it is also the thing I am criticised about the most.

I always say "Look after your wellbeing because you're going to need it. Prioritise it, understand its value and defend it".

These times away from my family and my work have been labelled 'selfish' and 'self-indulgent' by some. I will never apologise for prioritising this investment in my wellbeing. Obviously, from my busy work schedule and raft of commitments, it is almost impossible to keep up with and maintain the level of energy and passion my unique government leadership position and my family deserves. I am scheduled all day, every day and travel often. My diary directs me to where I need to be, when I can eat, how I am going to get there, where to park and often, when to take travel sick tablets. Each meeting requires an active representation of myself and my organisation. I am never passive in meetings, nor would I ever dream that is my job to do so. This is a life and a role that I absolutely love. However, as with every good engine or machine which needs to continue to perform with the same level of output, intensity, and credibility, I need some maintenance. As I get older, I need this more regularly, with daily tune-ups now being required. This doesn't have to be an expensive exercise. I do not need to take regular medication or have ongoing naps during the day. My need is about harnessing my energy to get ready for the next daily schedule of events and activities. To do this, I am clearly in need of some unscheduled, quiet, non-active brain activity. I need an hour where I do not make a decision, where I do not clear or read any briefs and I do not resolve conflicts. In this time, I don't want to be predetermined in any way, but rather some time to be flexible and responsive to what my brain, my body and my emotions need. Pilates and walking are it. This has taken me a very long time to understand my life, my needs and how I energise best. I love my downtime. It suits me.

In the end, it will ensure my family has a balanced and supportive mother at home, my workplace will receive a highly engaged, enthusiastic, and passionate leader and my abundant positive energy will hopefully spill over and influence the world around me. I want nothing less from my exercise and I feel it's working. Of course, by no means am I wishing this regime onto anyone else. I am only hoping for acceptance in my quest to protect my wellbeing, to build my sense of strength and to defend it. I am actually quite relentless about it. You should be too. You will need to find what works for you and be strong in your understanding of why this is important to you and the people around you. It's just a small part of my health and wellbeing, but often the most important. I feel that I'm finally starting to understand that.

According to the World Health Organisation "Health is a state of complete physical, mental and social wellbeing and not merely the absence of disease or infirmity".[65] This definition was part of a constitution that was published and agreed in New York in 1946. It still stands today.

So, I ask you "who feels they are in this constant state of complete physical, mental and social healthiness every day?". I ask that question at many of my presentations (often to women) and I still have not seen a single hand raised in agreement.

During the presentation, I also always ask who currently takes time out to build and strengthen their own wellbeing, whatever it is they choose to protect it with. Again, no hands.

At the end of each presentation, I also ask "who in this room will take time for their own health and wellbeing into the future?" which is always met by a sea of raised hands. This has always fascinated and troubled me at the same time as it tells me several things:

1. People do have an awareness of what actual health and wellbeing might be.
2. People do have an awareness that their health and wellbeing isn't good. In fact, I believe this applies to at least half of all adults.
3. People are not consciously choosing to do anything about it, or they simply can't or feel too overwhelmed to try, which also applies to about half of us.

What worries me is that I still hear "why do so many people today have mental health issues? In my day, we didn't have any of it. We had to be strong and push on. Nothing has changed". I am here to tell you; these comments are not valid. Things have changed and people are now starting to understand more about the reasons why. I want to reassure those who feel their mental health is being challenged that you are not alone, you are not weak and most likely, this is not your fault. Your feelings are shared by so many others and the research proves this. As a community, we definitely have a problem.

Firstly, I would like to introduce you to the term 'trauma' and how this often progresses to 'generational trauma'.

"Trauma is an experience of extreme stress or shock that is/or was, at some point, part of life. Traumatic events are often life-threatening and include natural disasters, motor vehicle accidents, sexual assault, difficult childbirth experiences or a pandemic. Any event that involves exposure to actual or threatened death, serious injury or sexual violence, has the potential to be traumatic. The trauma experienced can be physical and/or mental and not everyone will respond in the same way".[66]

Most of us (3 out of 4) have experienced this. More notably, most of our children (about 2 in 3) have experienced at least one traumatic event by the age of 17 years.[66] The experience of a traumatic event, the number of traumatic events and the type of traumatic events often impact us so much more than we realise. You may hear the term ACEs to describe these experiences. This stands for Adverse Childhood Experiences and the research shows, the more you have, the more likely you will be affected and will need support. Further, ACEs can increase the onset of mental illness and also the responses, or lack of, to treatment.[67]

Before I go on, I need to address some of these issues with reference to the stolen generation for Aboriginal and Torres Strait Islander families. There are two very important facts that I am not sure we all appreciate.

1. Forced removal policies were only ruled out in 1972. That's not that long ago! At that time, around one in ten, or 11 per cent of our precious Indigenous children, reported being taken from their families.[68]
2. The research has shown that this cohort of Australian children have been three times more likely to have been incarcerated in the last five years, 1.8 times more likely

to rely on government payments as their main source of income and 1.7 times more likely to experience violence, compared to those who were not removed.[68]

Again, I write this section, not to remind us about some of our shameful history as this is exactly what it is, but to ensure understanding of our environment, how this has impacted so many of our fellow Australians and continues to, for multiple generations in the past and sadly, more to come in the future. Our neighbours, our family, our friends are included here and we have to stop the cycle. These statistics will never progress us as a community. Enough.

Generational trauma, put simply, is when the descendants of people who have lived experience of traumatic events that have impacted their lives, feel similar adverse reactions and stress.[69]

What is difficult to understand is that there is no one size fits all to this.

Reactions vary by generation but often result in a heightened sense of vulnerability and helplessness, low self-esteem, depression, suicidality, substance abuse, dissociation, hypervigilance, intrusive thoughts, difficulty with relationships and attachment to others, difficulty in regulating aggression and extreme reactivity to stress.[69] This can affect us in so many ways and often, in all ways, often impacting our day-to-day functioning. "The exact mechanisms on how and why this occurs is not well understood but it is known to affect relationship skills, beliefs, attitudes which in turn, impacts someone's life followed closely by the life of future generations".[69]

If there is one thing I want you to get out of this difficult and quite emotional section, it is that these events are not your fault, they are extensive and all-encompassing. You need to be reminded that you are not alone, and you need to feel validated that it is likely, these events, whatever they might be, have affected you, your families and your children. However, this does not mean you can and should do nothing about it or that you can do nothing to recover and heal. A major step I would recommend for you is to understand what is really occurring around you. By understanding your current and previous environments, you will start to appreciate how much is actually working against you. You will understand the barriers that prevent you achieving good health and this will be so liberating. The second step is to understand how your village will get you through, and it can. This will be different for all of us. However, by knowledge, you will be better equipped on what and how to do things differently. Who to listen to, when to listen and when to make up your own mind. Question everything, challenge everything and listen differently.

In this next section, I am going to highlight some worrying facts about the wellbeing of specific groups within the communities in which we live. Our families, our neighbours, our friends. To be clear, this is not to categorise or generalise health and outcomes. Rather, it is to take a moment to understand some of the challenges unique to populations. Although I acknowledge, these are not the only people who need support, I know most about the challenges that impact priority populations uniquely. I write about these groups because I feel I can contribute most by concentrating on the population needs which can achieve great benefit.

Wellbeing and women

That said, in all my roles, experiences and professional and personal journeys, the wellbeing of women continues to concern me. When I was first appointed as the new Chief Executive Officer for Health and Welling Queensland, a close friend of mine reminded me it was my duty and my job to drive a strong leadership agenda for women. This was not to 'man-bash' or to make the current generation of males accountable for the decline in women's pay-gap and economic position, but rather to show that women can and should be leaders while they enjoy their good health, strong marriages, and family connections. I was quite surprised that someone was actually saying this, that there was a need for such a conscious and deliberate agenda. My eyes have been wide-open since. I would go as far as to say it is rare to find a woman in an intense leadership position who is working, maintaining good social connections, enjoying wonderful partnerships with family and friends, feels empowered to make decisions, is balanced and supported by strong mental health. In most cases, some of these areas suffer to ensure success in others. Whilst I don't think you can have everything, I strongly believe you can manipulate and manage your environment towards helping women rather than hindering them in their path, whether it be through a career, motherhood, social connections or just simply life.

Wellbeing and men

It is well accepted that men's overall health in Australia is good. Globally, men experience a good life expectancy (80.4 years) as Australia celebrates being one of only 12 countries where this figure exceeds 80 years of age.[70] However, through the life course, men struggle with challenges that appear to be somewhat unique to their gender.

Boys, 5-14 years, experience significant issues of asthma and anxiety. These are the highest cause of health burden for this age group.[70]

As boys mature, the pressure of adolescence presents new challenges of peer influence and risk-taking activities and behaviours which can challenge healthy choices and overall health outcomes. It is important to note that the adolescent brain does not mature until the mid-20s. Worryingly, from the ages of 15-24 years, self-inflicting injuries and suicide rates rise as well as alcohol-use. This seems to worsen again in males aged 25-44 years, along with an increase in back problems. At older age groups, senior men, aged over 85 years have the highest rates of suicide across Australia.[70] So what's going wrong?

If you think men are most reluctant to ask for help, you'd be right, however, overall, this has improved and is still improving. Women are much more likely to access timely healthcare, however, the gap between the genders is improving.[70]

Although most men generally report seeing a health professional at least once in the past year, it is now reported that men tend to seek help with shorter consultations or wait until their condition is advanced, often preventing an opportunity for effective early detection and treatment. Saying that, most men (approximately ¾) don't seek help for mental health when they need it.[70]

What is most concerning to me is that many young men report experiencing a mental health condition or symptoms in their lives and often do nothing about it. Suicide is more than three times more common in males than females and twice as common in Aboriginal and Torres Strait Islander males, as non-Indigenous males.[70] It is crystal clear that men require much more than what is provided via their physical medical appointments; which are rare and annual at best. What more should we and could we be providing to men of all ages, to ensure we look after their mental and physical health?

Clearly, our environment is not set up adequately to support good mental health for men across all ages.

Wellbeing and young people

If there's one thing that stands out most commonly from all of my thousands of patient consultations, it is the level of acceptance of bullying among children, parents and families.

Examples of statements made in my clinics that have truly stunned and saddened me includes:

"He's not called the bad words anymore – just tank and fridge, so that's better".

"We're all big boned and that's how the school accepts us".

"The school has better things to do than to worry about name-calling".

"We've all been bullied – throughout our whole family".

What's worse, it appears that often nobody had queried or questioned these statements. Rather, their city had accepted this as reality and something that simply cannot be changed.

What concerns me is that I don't see this improving. In fact, it's getting worse and obtaining good, credible statistics is difficult. This is a problem in itself.

One Australian study estimated that most children (70%) in their teenage years have been 'bullied' at least once in the past 12 months.[71] My feeling is that it's worse than the statistics are telling us. However, *why* the statistics representing this incredibly important issue are not well understood or measured, is the bigger issue for me.

We all know that bullying can lead to a wide range of adverse physical, mental, social and emotional impacts on our youth.[72] The good news is that in Australia, schools are improving. In fact, some primary schools are actively implementing targeted interventions which have proven to reduce the incidence of bullying.[73,74]

My advice here is to lean into your children and your schools around bullying. There is a lot of awareness in Australia about the issue and I can see change afoot. Children need to be reminded of their worth and value, to arm and protect them against the effects of bullying (and cyberbullying) when it occurs.

To be clear, this section is telling us that bullying of children impacts them on many levels, with the long-term effects varying. However, schools in Australia are starting to understand this, but they will need students and parents to report on what is happening to them first-hand.

A better surveillance system of monitoring incidence and other aspects of bullying is urgently required. This will allow us to best understand and more importantly, explain what bullying is actually doing in our environments.[72] Ultimately, prevention, healing and potentially eradication of future trauma for our future generations, especially those already feeling vulnerable, will be promoted.

It's not your fault!

Wellbeing and seniors

I am embarrassed to say that it wasn't until the release of the 2021 report – the Royal Commission into Aged Care Quality and Safety, that I truly understood the sheer ignorance in our society of the wellbeing of our critically important seniors. These are the holders of our stories, our memories, the history of our nation, our society and our journey through famine, war, depression, and life. Yet, they have not been dignified with the respect and care they afforded to us through providing the basic requirements for life in their senior years. They took the future of the next generations seriously. They made a commitment to us that our freedom would be protected, and they delivered. I am sad and disappointed with the outcomes of this report and want to outline some very important facts about the wellbeing of our most precious historians – our seniors.

We are aging as a population. In 2017, an estimated 15 per cent of Australians were classed as 'older' compared to 13 per cent reported a decade earlier.[75] By 'older' here, we are referring to Australians aged older than 65 years. We know that the majority (95%) of older people lived in their own home, with the remainder in residential aged care facilities.

For our seniors, many are already lonely.

Loneliness has been linked to premature death, poor physical and mental health and general dissatisfaction with life.[76] "In our seniors, it is well known that those who are married report the lowest levels of loneliness". Of course, I'm not saying that we all need to go out and get married, however, there is a lesson in this. People who have their supportive village, will be less lonely and will improve their wellbeing. In turn, this may actually even extend the length of their lives. For both men and women, those who are married are likely to live two years longer than their unmarried counterparts.

Research shows that in our senior years, reducing loneliness reduces depression.[77] However, our environments often don't support this to happen. According to a research study in 2022, major barriers for older people in forming social connections arise from the restrictions of reduced physical mobility and chronic health issues, difficulties accessing appropriate transport, digital exclusion, reduced self-confidence and self-efficacy, financial concerns about the cost of activities, limited mental health literacy and the enduring stigma surrounding mental illness, loneliness and social isolation.[77] For older people experiencing chronic loneliness, there are serious health consequences. These effects are known to increase the risk of death more than significant public health issues, such as smoking and obesity.[77]

Differing from bullying in young people, the association between loneliness and social isolation and poor mental health, is well understood.

Keeping ourselves well connected physically, emotionally, and mentally is key. However, the environment often doesn't support us to do this, even though we understand the research. Approximately half of all older adults in Australia have a chronic disease, impairing our ability to engage with our village.[78]

To be clear, this simply shows that our community and our villages are so important. This can take many forms including marriage, partnerships, community groups, family groups, gender groups or even just the ability to stroll through the shopping centre every day. All these help.

A connected and engaged village wards off loneliness when we get it right.

Wellbeing and workforces

I am pleased to say I am starting to see our wellbeing be considered and even prioritised in the workforce. However, I am also deeply conscious that the support of our workforce within the current environment post-COVID-19 is sporadic and fragile, yet the impacts of getting this right are proven and strong.

Health is distributed unequally by occupation. Workers on a lower rung of the occupational ladder report worse health, have a higher probability of disability and die earlier than workers higher up the occupational hierarchy. Studies show health status monotonically improves with higher levels of occupation: 81 per cent of elementary workers report good or very good health as opposed to 90 per cent of those in high-level and university-level occupations.[79]

Working in a satisfactory job environment improves self-reported health and reduces limitations in activities of daily living.[79]

With the COVID-19 pandemic placing a significant burden on all individuals across the globe, healthcare workers appeared to be among the hardest hit. Responding directly to the pandemic, while also treating non-COVID-19 patients, caring for their families and their own health, high rates of burnout, psychological stress and sadly even suicide, have been shown among our healthcare workforce.[80] According to the 2021 Census data, one in seven people in the Australian workforce are working in the health care and social assistance industry.[81] My question here is – are we doing enough to look after them?

Queensland unemployment rates are at an all-time low. Although this sounds wonderful, it has impacts of its own that require management and planning. Queensland's unemployment rate was 3.8 per cent as at March 2023[82] which means only 110, 216 Queenslanders remain unemployed, compared to nearly 30,000 more in 2013.[83] Any current employer knows we need to keep our workforces well, happy and engaged. This makes sense, however, it's not just for the benefit of the employees, it's to actually keep the economy going.

"Non-communicable diseases account for 38 million deaths each year. With more than a half of the world's population spending one third of their adult lives at work, workplace wellness programs have been identified as a strategy to tackle non-communicable diseases".[84] In addition to this, research tells us by "improving the health and wellbeing of workers, productivity, corporate performance and community prosperity also improve".[85]

Looking after our own families (whether home or work families) is not difficult and it should be top priority for all of us. I wanted to share with you seven top strategies published from the National Institute of Health, United States of America when referring to our precious healthcare workforce:[80]

1. Access to mental health resources should be immediate and individualised.
2. Short- and long-term individualised wellness and mental health interventions should be developed to address both the physical and emotional tolls of COVID-19.
3. Wellness for the healthcare workforce should be optimised

with the implementation of individual and organisational strategies, across the areas of nutrition, exercise, mindfulness, sleep quality and reducing burnout.

4. Quality and accessible personal protective equipment should be provided for all healthcare workers, to ensure security and to reduce the likelihood of infection for themselves and their loved ones.

5. The opportunity to research and implement telehealth should be used in a variety of settings, to limit exposure to infection.

6. Stigma associated with mental health symptoms and the psychological impact of significant stressful events should be reduced among healthcare workers.

7. Participation in new healthcare workforce community groups should be encouraged to facilitate connections and reduce feelings of isolation.

To me, these set minimum standards. You should just implement these. However, we should also consider what's most relevant to you and the people you work with right now in addition to the basics. There is nothing basic about workforce stress in 2024. For my workforce, it's about purpose and having fun. I would add three more to make it a top ten (noting no science or evidence behind this, but learnings from my own experience) …

8. Reassure your workforce with evidence of the impact they are making for their patients, consumers or communities. A sense of purpose builds such resilience and the proof of what they are doing is even better.

9. Enjoy what you do. Make sure there is laugher and joy every day in whatever it is you are working on. Stay strong, but also humble. Celebrate the successes, but also be bold enough to acknowledge and learn from the failures.

10. Provide the leadership through 'walking the walk' as your critical workforce is watching every single thing you do. They need a strong leader, one who is willing to take care of themselves, as well as others.

Wellbeing and weight stigma

I will start this section by saying, weight stigma should never be tolerated. The name-calling, the judgement, the trolling, the social media shaming and the imagery impacts, not only on our wellbeing but our health as a society. If we were performing a health check on our population right now based on the impact of weight stigma in the current environment, we would fail and go straight to the intervention. So that's what I'm doing. Let's understand weight stigma and then let's influence and shape our community to be one with zero tolerance to what this issue attracts.

Who has been affected by weight stigma? The answer is – most of us, either directly or indirectly and it's got to stop.

The idea of weight stigma has always worried me. The one thing that I remember clearly from my clinics over the past 20 years is how weight stigma manifests itself. There are just so many ways. It is pervasive, debilitating and everywhere.

Weight stigma can be described as "discrimination towards an individual due to their size and weight".[86] In my experience, it manifests itself differently through gender and age. Calling a young adolescent male 'tank' or 'fridge' as they played football appeared to be more tolerated than calling young women 'stinky' or 'fat'. Making fun of older teenagers and young adult men for not being big enough to play footy or to make the swim team, is also common. I'm here to tell you all of it is wrong, it's intentional and it hurts.

"Weight stigma is the consequence of weight bias, which is the negative belief associated with living in a larger body. Weight stigmatisation can occur across many different environments including school, the workplace, healthcare settings, personal relationships and the media. Teasing, social exclusion, physical assault, negative body language and environments not accommodating for people living in a bigger body, are all examples of weight stigmatisation".[86] The worst experiences for me were when my younger patients didn't want to talk about the subject of weight stigma in front of their parents, as they somehow felt they let their families down. This still goes on today and I am here to tell you, that would never be tolerated in my clinics. Empowering these children, parents and families to not only understand, but to influence their environments back, is key.

Weight stigma presents as one of the most common forms of discrimination among adults and one of the most prevalent forms of bullying among children.[87] It should be of no surprise that research suggests a strong association between weight stigma and poor mental health, in addition to the promotion of health behaviours that perpetuate poor health and obesity including binge eating, increased food consumption, the avoidance of physical activity, physiological stress and weight gain.[87] Astounding research in the US has found individuals experiencing weight discrimination exhibit a 60 per cent greater risk of dying, irrespective of their body mass index (BMI).[88] Chronic social stress resulting in the dysregulation of metabolic health and inflammation are believed to be the mechanisms underlying this increased risk.[88]

I say 'ENOUGH'. Our children are amazing and need to be reminded of it.

WHAT THIS MEANS FOR YOUR VILLAGE:

Our wellbeing is paramount to every single part of our life. Make sure you take the time to consider your own wellbeing, be selfish about it, prioritise it and adhere to it every single day. Your wellbeing is your health. Look after your wellbeing. Protect and defend it, because you're going to need it.

Chapter 4 References

1. World Health Organisation. 2023. *Constitution* [Online]. WHO. Available: https://www.who.int/about/governance/constitution [Accessed 2023].
2. Australian Institute of Health and Welfare. 2022. *Mental Health Services in Australia: Stress and Trauma* [Online]. AIHW. Available: https://www.aihw.gov.au/reports/mental-health-services/stress-and-trauma [Accessed 2023].
3. Hughes, K., Lowey, H., Quigg, Z. & Bellis, M. A. 2016. Relationships between adverse childhood experiences and adult mental well-being: results from an English national household survey. *BMC Public Health,* 16, 222.
4. Australian Institute of Health and Welfare. 2018. *New report shows long-term disadvantage for Australia's Stolen Generations* [Online]. AIHW. Available: https://www.aihw.gov.au/news-media/media-releases/2018/august/new-report-shows-long-term-disadvantage-for-austra [Accessed 2023].
5. American Psychological Association. 2023. *Intergenerational trauma* [Online]. Available: https://dictionary.apa.org/intergenerational-trauma [Accessed 2023].
6. Department of Health. 2019. *National Men's Health Strategy 2020-2030* [Online]. Australian Government. Available: https://www.health.gov.au/sites/default/files/documents/2021/05/national-men-s-health-strategy-2020-2030_0.pdf [Accessed 2023].
7. Australian Institute of Health and Welfare. 2022. *Bullying* [Online]. AIHW. Available: https://www.aihw.gov.au/reports/children-youth/australias-children/contents/justice-and-safety/bullying [Accessed 2023].

8. Jadambaa, A., Thomas, H. J., Scott, J. G., Graves, N., Brain, D. & Pacella, R. 2019. Prevalence of traditional bullying and cyberbullying among children and adolescents in Australia: A systematic review and meta-analysis. *Australian & New Zealand Journal of Psychiatry,* 53, 878-888.

9. Department of Education. 2023. *Bullying and cyberbullying - preventing and responding* [Online]. Australian Government. Available: https://behaviour.education.qld.gov.au/supporting-student-behaviour/bullying-and-cyberbullying [Accessed 2023].

10. Queensland Government. 2018. *Queensland ramps up action on bullying* [Online]. Available: https://statements.qld.gov.au/statements/83941 [Accessed 2023].

11. Australian Institute of Health and Welfare. 2017. *Aging and welfare* [Online]. AIHW. Available: https://www.aihw.gov.au/getmedia/d18a1d2b-692c-42bf-81e2-47cd54c51e8d/aihw-australias-welfare-2017-chapter5-1.pdf.aspx [Accessed 2023].

12. Australian Institute of Health and Welfare. 2021. *Social isolation and loneliness* [Online]. AIHW. Available: https://www.aihw.gov.au/reports/australias-welfare/social-isolation-and-loneliness-covid-pandemic [Accessed 2023].

13. Thompson C, M. D., Bird S 2022. Evaluation of the Improving Social Connectedness of Older Australians project pilot: Informing future policy considerations. *In:* CENTRE FOR HEALTH SERVICE DEVELOPMENT & INSTITUTE, Australian Health Services Research Institute (eds.). University of Wollongong.

14. Australian Institute of Health and Welfare. 2022. *Chronic conditions and multimorbidity* [Online]. AIHW. Available: https://www.aihw.gov.au/reports/australias-health/chronic-conditions-and-multimorbidity [Accessed 2023].

15. Ravesteijn, B., Van Kippersluis, H. & Van Doorslaer, E. 2013. The contribution of occupation to health inequality. *Res Econ Inequal,* 21, 311-332.

16. Shreffler, J., Petrey, J. & Huecker, M. 2020. The Impact of COVID-19 on Healthcare Worker Wellness: A Scoping Review. *West J Emerg Med,* 21, 1059-1066.

17. Australian Bureau of Statistics. 2022. *A caring nation – 15 per cent of Australia's workforce in Health Care and Social Assistance industry* [Online]. ABS. Available: https://www.abs.gov.au/media-centre/media-releases/caring-nation-15-cent-australias-workforce-health-care-and-social-assistance-industry [Accessed 2023].

18. The Queensland Cabinet and Ministerial Directory. 2023. *Queensland's low unemployment continues* [Online]. Available: https://statements.qld.gov.au/statements/97559#:~:text=Queensland's%20trend%20unemployment%20rate%20was,state's%20strong%20labour%20market%20performance [Accessed 2023].

19. Queensland Treasury. 2023. *Economy, Labour and Employment (State)* [Online]. Queensland Government Statistician's Office. Available: https://www.qgso.qld.gov.au/statistics/theme/economy/labour-employment/state [Accessed 2023].

20. Zacharias, K. D., Hundal, N., Kumar, S., Shigematsu, L. M. R., Bahl, D. & Wipfli, H. 2019. Corporate Wellness Programs: Promoting a Healthy Workforce. *In:* WITHERS,

M. & MCCOOL, J. (eds.) *Global Health Leadership: Case Studies From the Asia-Pacific.* Cham: Springer International Publishing.

21. Pronk, N. P. 2019. Public health, business, and the shared value of workforce health and wellbeing. *Lancet Public Health,* 4, e323.

22. World Obesity. 2022. *Weight Stigma* [Online]. Available: https://www.worldobesity.org/what-we-do/our-policy-priorities/weight-stigma [Accessed 2023].

23. Puhl, R. & Suh, Y. 2015. Health Consequences of Weight Stigma: Implications for Obesity Prevention and Treatment. *Current Obesity Reports,* 4, 182-190.

24. Tomiyama, A. J., Carr, D., Granberg, E. M., Major, B., Robinson, E., Sutin, A. R. & Brewis, A. 2018. How and why weight stigma drives the obesity 'epidemic' and harms health. *BMC Med,* 16, 123.

CHAPTER 5

What's coming?

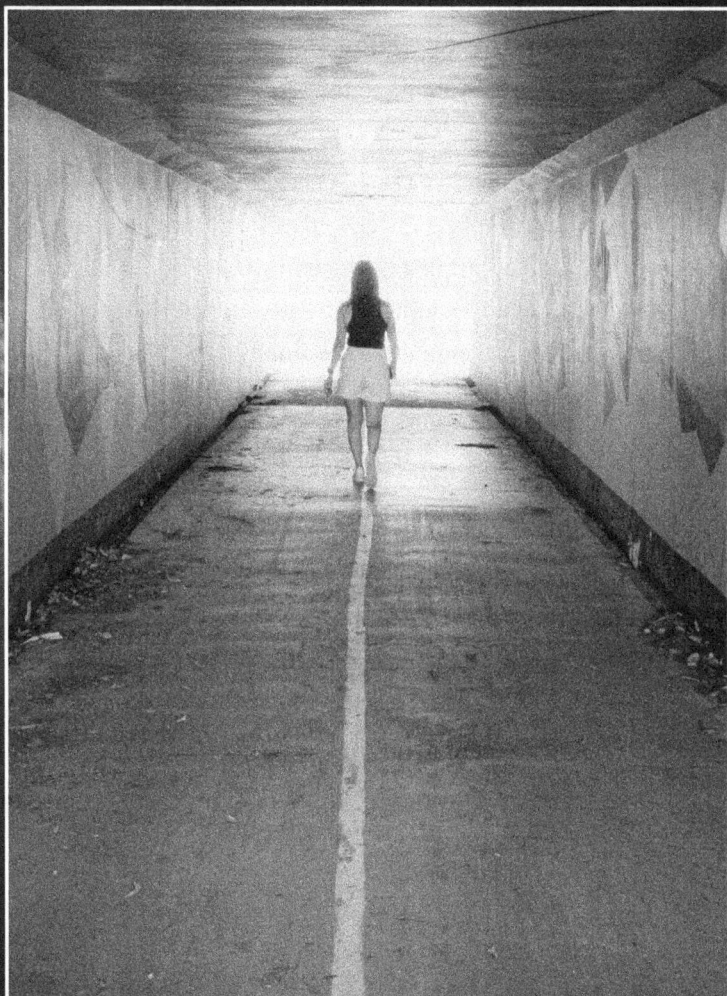

CHAPTER 5

What's coming?

With all this new information, it may not be of much comfort to know that so much more is coming. In my opinion, it is always good to understand, even at a very basic level, some of the mega trends that can impact all of us into the future. I have had the privilege of being at many planning events, launches and meetings, where many of these topics have been discussed as they have progressed from idea to project to sustainable focus for government. From this information, I have to admit that I am so positive about our future. I see what our communities are finally focussing on and investing in, and it's right.

However, the inherent problem with all of these big 'megatrends' is that many of us don't understand them, the link to our health, our communities and the future of our children. I am going to try to help with making those connections as I have had the luxury of time and space for consideration.

In the past, through my experiences in the world of academia, industry and government, I am always aware that we are sometimes so insular in our communication, events and reporting that we often forget to let the rest of the world know what we are doing or, even worse, we forget to ask people whether this was even important to them. Yet we continue on, patting ourselves on the back and progressing the narrative in the often, isolated circles of networks that exist. I see this equally occurring globally. There are many documents where the term 'megatrend' is used, usually through a forecasting event where large consultancy and academic institutions predict the changes in the future. The definition of 'megatrend' is a major movement, pattern or trend emerging in the macroenvironment. I want to explain my top megatrends below:

1. Wellbeing Economy
2. Food insecurity
3. Equity
4. Walkability
5. Data
6. Climate change
7. Women
8. Parenting
9. Leadership
10. Social media

A very big thankyou to Health and Wellbeing Queensland for allowing me to include these narratives in my book. Although I authored these and published these as blogs, they belong to Health and Wellbeing Queensland[89] and I applaud the leadership and understanding by allowing me to add these for the greater good. Please enjoy them.

1. Wellbeing Economy

You may have heard in media channels, newspapers or on the news, the introduction of a Wellbeing Economy as we plan and forecast our federal budget. For clarity, a wellbeing economy is designed to serve people and the planet. It's as simple as that. However, I have heard many people, including my own parents, reporting their frustration at the discussion. The term is brand new to this country and is not well understood. Again, this appears another failure of our current environment. In the race to publish articles, announcements, and investment commitments, even when we remain evidence-based and safe, we often forget to tell a story and take a community along the journey. In fact, for many of us living within the same isolated circles, we have already heard about these megatrends and other future considerations that are on our horizon. Many of us feel very comfortable we understand the concepts of the future including the Wellbeing Economy, however, I don't feel this is the majority, as communicating the journey to our population is often omitted.

Countries such as New Zealand, Finland, Iceland, Scotland, Wales and the United States have either already implemented a Wellbeing Economy or are well on the way. They see the value of measuring factors other than their gross domestic product (GDP) or money. In fact, GDP is a country's monetary measure. When we talk about a Wellbeing Economy, we are adding conditions beyond money and moving towards creating conditions in which people improve their health and wellbeing to thrive. This is exactly in line with what this book is asking for. My sense is that the introduction of the Wellbeing Economy in Australia is a very good thing. It's not a 'yoga wellness retreat'. Other countries are quite advanced now in making progress and providing outcomes, that are so much more than just money that we need to focus on. The Wellbeing Economy does exactly that.

In our social system as we understand more about what truly affects our health, we accept social conditions that sit outside of health which often affect our health the most. This includes education, housing, transport and food, as well as economic growth.

I was reading the news last week and came across an excellent story that showcased the following survey. I think this clearly shows what a Wellbeing Economy can achieve and just how important it is to our population. I just don't think we feel empowered enough to understand it for what it is.

A recent study of Australians asked participants, *"Given what you know about the state of the world and your own financial situation, is it absolutely your highest priority to become twice as wealthy in the next 20 years and consume twice as much?"*. **Very few people respond in the affirmative.** Those who do see it as desirable still usually rank it below other goals such as staying healthy, having satisfying work, being in a strong relationship, feeling secure in their neighbourhood and seeing children happy.[90]

This is proof we all want a Wellbeing Economy, to allow us to work together in improving the social, mental health, societal and physical factors within our environment that affect our health. However, as a country, we still don't really know what it is.

Looking to an example, in 2019, New Zealand implemented its first Wellbeing Budget, a commitment to placing population wellbeing and the environment at the heart of all policies. The design principles to support the Wellbeing Budget include: working across government to assess, develop and implement policies that improve wellbeing; focussing on the needs of the current population whilst also considering long-term impacts for future generations and tracking the Government's progress with broader measures of success including the health of the country's finances, natural resources, people and communities.[91] As an example, this means schools and hospitals receive ongoing funding to support families and most importantly, the Wellbeing Budget is non-negotiable.[92]

2.   Food Insecurity

Food insecurity is not well understood in Australia, yet nearly one-third of us living in remote areas experience it. Despite a lack of national data, we know the numbers are significant in urban, regional and rural areas too.

When people think of the term 'food insecurity', they often jump to the food shortages of the depression era or to children in developing countries. For many of us, the lack of fresh, healthy food available to all Queenslanders doesn't immediately spring to mind. But why?

When a person is unable to feed themselves and their family nutritious food to meet their dietary needs and preferences

– in whatever form that takes – they are characterised as experiencing food insecurity. This exists on a spectrum and includes worry and anxiety about future meals.

Too many households experience food insecurity and it's getting worse.

Too many Australians do not know where their next meal is coming from. Despite the efforts of government and community-controlled sectors, this problem has persisted, due to its sheer complexity and the impact on the social determinants (including housing and economic security).

National surveillance of food security measures is limited, with the most recent data showing 31 per cent of people living in remote areas experience food insecurity, compared to four per cent of the general population.

Add a pandemic to the mix and food insecurity is a dire and real issue for many. Queenslanders who were struggling before COVID-19, are going hungry more often now. Three in 10 Australians experiencing food insecurity in 2020 had not gone hungry before the pandemic.

The nation's cost-of-living crisis has also hit our eating habits, as prices for fresh produce soar at the supermarket. In 2024, we are seeing the impact across our nation.

New data from the Fruit & Vegetable Consortium, an alliance focused on boosting vegetable consumption, revealed affordability as the top reason Queenslanders were not eating enough vegetables for good health.[93]

In the national survey of more than 1000 grocery shoppers, 85 per cent of regional Queenslanders and 72 per cent of shoppers in the state's capital linked vegetables becoming more expensive to not eating enough greens.

An issue compounded by shame and stigma.

Unsurprisingly, the guilt and shame associated with not having enough food is compounded by stigma. Often, families do not ask for help. Coping strategies include adults prioritising children's meals over their own; forgoing other essentials to afford food; or skipping meals. It can manifest in overeating when food is available to prepare for times of scarcity and can include a diet of 'cheaper' energy-dense, nutrition-poor foods, which ultimately contributes to unhealthy weight and chronic disease.

These actions can be misinterpreted as 'making unhealthy choices'. However, they are actually deliberate acts to save money, avoid the stigma associated with asking for help and feed one's family, when the healthy choice isn't available.

For First Nations Australians living outside metropolitan areas, the situation is dire, with 28 per cent of those living in remote communities experiencing problems with their household facilities, preventing safe food storage, preparation and consumption. One in five households in very remote areas do not have the facilities needed to enable food security.

A vicious cycle of food insecurity and chronic disease.

Those who do not have the ability to buy, prepare and store healthy food because their circumstances do not allow, also face poorer health outcomes. Poor nutrition contributes to 62 per cent of coronary heart disease burden, 41 per cent of type 2 diabetes burden and 34 per cent of stroke burden. Diet is the leading risk factor for cardiovascular disease, which is the number one cause of death for First Nations Australians living in remote areas. High BMI is the leading risk factor for burden of disease in remote First Nations communities, and this burden is almost double in remote areas compared to major cities.

Our food system is not secure, with remote areas hit hardest.

Remote communities often rely on one general store for food. Sparse food outlets are not well connected to homes via public transport and families may need to walk long distances or use personal transport (if available), which incurs extra fuel costs. Due to barriers – including freight, distance and supply-chain coordination – basic food items are less available in remote stores. It has been documented that 12 per cent of basic healthy food basket items are missing from very remote stores.

The cost of freight to remote areas of Australia is thought to contribute up to 20 per cent of the cost of food in these areas. This is even higher for remote Island communities. A healthy food basket is 20 per cent and 31 per cent higher in remote and very remote areas (respectively) compared to urban centres, with the price of a healthy food basket up to 50 per cent higher in Cape York compared to Brisbane. In Queensland, families need to spend 23 per cent of their income to achieve the Australian Guide to Healthy Eating recommended diet. In very remote areas, this rises to 35 per cent of the median household income – rendering a healthy diet unaffordable.

Compounding the problem is the First Nations employment rate, which was 49 per cent compared to 75 per cent for non-Indigenous Australians, in 2018. In very remote areas, the unemployment rate for First Nations people (15-64 years) is double that of major cities (29% versus 15%). This is the result of inequitable employment and training opportunities in rural and remote regions.

For me personally, it's about understanding this is a truly wicked problem in Queensland and Australia and if you're feeling the pinch right now, you are not alone. You certainly haven't done anything wrong.

3. Equity

As a dietitian, I used to think if I studied hard, worked relentlessly and provided the best evidence-based nutritional management to my patients, I could solve the problem of obesity.

I equipped all my patients with every piece of information on eating plans, meals and resources to support a healthy diet for their household, accompanied by the best physical activity advice. I reviewed patients regularly, communicated well and congratulated all the wins (small and big) to ensure they remained on track. I didn't always succeed. So what was missing from my approach? I didn't take equity into account.

What does that even mean and why don't we teach our health graduates about equity?

In Australia, obesity is lowest among people who have a tertiary qualification and highest among those who have not finished high school. People living outside major cities and people renting their homes or paying off a mortgage, are more likely to be overweight or obese than others.

We know obesity rates are disproportionately higher among those experiencing disadvantage and therefore, long-term gains in reducing obesity will require understanding why this is so. How can we better understand the relationship between level of disadvantage and health outcomes, to better address these upstream factors?

In retrospect, it is clear that despite my good intentions, I was missing parts of the picture. I didn't always consider my patient as someone who lives within, and is affected by, environments and systems that influence how they behave, how they are perceived and what they have access to. I was asking patients who already experience disadvantage some of the time to work against all the powerful influences that surround them, with many factors outside of their control. In other words, I was fixing up patients only to send them back to the same environments that promoted the obesity in the first place.

This is a major systems issue and challenge for governments and communities globally. A significant amount of practice and research over the past two decades demonstrates such disparities across a range of health outcomes, as well as a growing body of evidence highlighting the importance of addressing the social determinants of health – that is, the circumstances in which we are born, grow up, live, work and age. These circumstances are shaped by economic, social and political forces. It is now widely acknowledged that achieving equity in health requires changing the odds in additional areas to health, such as education, work, employment, income and housing.

Examples of where inequity affects our health include:

- Having a secure home supports good health, employment and engagement with education. Not everyone has the same access to housing, with nearly 60 per cent of homeless people in Australia aged under 35, and 28 per cent being Aboriginal and Torres Strait Islander people.

- People with access to good education earn more money, live longer and are healthier. Yet, there is a 25 per cent gap in completing Year 12 between people from the highest and lowest socioeconomic backgrounds, and 40 per cent of people from the lowest socioeconomic backgrounds do not finish Year 12.

- People who are employed are healthier and healthy people are more likely to work. Beyond providing the income to allow for healthy lifestyle choices, employment can increase social capital, enhance psychological wellbeing and promote positive self-esteem.

We are each born into different circumstances and don't all have access to the same resources and opportunities. We do not all start from the same place. As a result, obesity, like a range of other poor health or life outcomes, is not experienced to the same extent or in the same way by all Queenslanders. Life is not fair, but we can do something about making it more equitable. Equity exists when social conditions enable communities, families and individuals to flourish. Working towards equity begins with acknowledging that current and historical social norms, and processes of power and decision-making have generated privilege and disparities. Achieving equity requires society working collectively to address and redress systemic disparities in power, resources, opportunities and participation.

We know obesity and health inequalities can affect the life expectancy of our next generation.

Striving for equity is an important moral goal, and it also makes economic sense. For example, it is suggested inequity in education costs Australia more than $118 billion across a six-year period. And conversely, policies to improve high school and tertiary education completion rates also improve GDP per capita.

Across Australia and Queensland, governments, community organisations, practitioners and advocacy groups in a wide array of sectors are fighting for equity within key areas such as housing, education, the criminal justice system, employment, income and workplaces. These efforts can be amplified if we recognise the interconnections between these drivers of inequity and synthesise them into a unified view with shared solutions.

It means we have to look at the systems differently – understand the impact they have on our lives, and how they interact with each other to create or prevent fair outcomes. Ultimately, addressing inequity requires undoing institutional and relational systemic barriers to achieving positive life outcomes. Systems leadership, which is about harnessing collective knowledge and bringing leaders together as catalysts for change, highlights the importance of working together to achieve this.

So, back to my patients. What I learned as I worked with my patients and families is that now, more than ever, we need to understand the environment our patients are living in and the impact it has on their lives. As clinicians, teachers, parents or public servants, we must work with others to integrate services to provide a tailored and holistic response that seeks to address the range of factors that influence people's lives.

Patients and families don't care about who owned what agenda previously. They expect us to do our jobs and right now, we need to focus on equity in Australia. It's having an impact and our environment must be in our sights to focus on.

4. Walkability

Put simply, 'walkability' is defined as the accessibility from where we live (our home) to where we need to get to (our work, shops, transport, schools and other amenities). The closer these facilities are to our starting base, the higher the walkability score. As we start to understand the impact of the social determinants of health, walkability of our 'village' clearly becomes critical to the quality of our lives. In fact, it can determine how much we walk (or ride or scooter) to schools, work, public transports, how much we use parks and green spaces and even how often we access the local supermarket. In turn all these things contribute to our health and wellbeing. Once I understood this, I made walkability a criterion when I purchased my family home and now, I use it when I choose somewhere to holiday. I know that if I can walk to a coffee shop and the walk is pleasant and safe, I will do it. I know that if I live within walking distance to my job, I will more likely walk or ride to get there. I know that if I live close enough to some of my friends, I will more likely have a social connection with them.

The other part of walkability that is critical to me is not just the proximity of all of these important things but also my acceptance of walking.

As I get older, I know walking is becoming more important to me, but I have never been able to articulate 'why'.

What I do know is that walking is something I now prioritise and value. It makes me feel good about myself as I start to become overwhelmed with a sense of energy, contentment, and happiness but in a very serene and calm way (which has never made sense to me).

I have always been a runner (albeit, slow and steady but very consistent and regular). I still love to run but I don't run the long distances anymore. A 30-minute run for me is adequate and helps clear my mind quickly, as this is what is needed sometimes.

Walking is different.

Appreciating the environment is something I am only starting to learn and appreciate, and it's having a very big impact on every part of my life. My favourite walk is one that is long, in the sun, at my own pace, through different tracks and paths and involves lots of scenery. It's amazing what you pick up when you walk. I know so much more about my local community and all it has to offer; from the small book exchange boxes to the gorgeous bush tracks (often in the middle of busy areas) to the small animals and the neighbouring dogs who say hello, I appreciate the diversity of what all of it has to offer (something you could never see, feel or experience in a car).

One of my favourite things to watch is either the sunrise or the sunset from the top of the hill I have just climbed and where I live, there are many. The colours of both events are magical and make me feel ridiculously good, something I never noticed through running.

We know that walking is the most popular form of physical recreation in Queensland, 30 minutes of walking each day actually improves your health and also improves mental health by reducing anxiety, depression, negative moods and improving self-esteem.[94]

I have recently started listening to podcasts and downloading audio books and listening through my ear pods. This is a new world for me and one that I have embraced fully. I love nothing better than having two hours to spend on my favourite walking tracks, supported by good shoes that will go the distance, my ear pods, my dog and a terrific book to listen to. It's a new experience and the experience I need sometimes. I am not in a rush and I often stop to take a closer look (again something I have never done before). The time flies.

My dog, Maggie, is a good reminder that I have to walk. It helps. The fact that she clearly loves it, supports the whole commitment. Just taking five steps towards the dog lead and my walking shoes creates excitement in my house.

I will make room for walking as it gives me back more to my mental health, physical health, emotional health than anything else in my life. I am so grateful I live in Queensland. Brisbane, the Gold Coast and Bribie Island are three favourite places to walk and I never book a holiday without access to these tracks. It's not what I like anymore, it's now what I need to continue to succeed in the life I lead every day.

Someone once told me it was *my* attachment to *my* country. The feeling of being at peace, grounded and of belonging is overwhelming.

I know walking will be a part of life for the rest of my life.

Sometimes I take it for granted. At the age of 50, I have no aches or pains. My body is able to support walking which makes me feel good in return. However, that's not the case for everyone.

Walking can be hard for the 900,000 Queenslanders who have a disability. With my Father requiring a power wheelchair for mobility, I am reminded of this every day. He has incomplete quadriplegia, but that doesn't stop him, nor should it.

All of those positive attributes and emotions I enjoy from walking should be afforded to everyone, regardless of physical ability. Recently, my family went for a day trip to Bribie Island. I have never seen my Dad as happy as when he is at the beach. I saw a complete mood change in my Dad that became obvious through his physical demeanour. The smells, the sun, the warm temperatures, the bush (leading along the beach tracks), the birds and wildlife and the ambience attracts the same magical feeling to Dad as he makes his way along the perfectly structured pathways (well done Bribie Island). When the kangaroos jumped out it was something else (seriously)!

Due to my Dad's requirements, we only visit places where I know will be safe, easy for Dad to get around and accessible to toilets and parking. Queensland is getting better, but we're not there yet.

Our checklist includes:

- The width of the path
- Gaps between and dividing pathways. Why do these even exist?

- Is it even? What is it made out of?

- Is there a gradient?

- Accessibility of toilets

- Accessibility of parking

- Accessibility into shopping centres or shops

- What do the lifts look like? Can they fit a power chair?

- What surface are the picnic tables?

- Can Dad's chair fit under the height of the tables?

- How windy is the area? Dad's temperature drops very quickly – will we need warmer blankets if there are no wind breakers in the area. We need extra gloves and socks often.

My family and I often talk through the impact of having a physical disability and the challenges people living with a disability face. My Father's comments are always brilliant as he starts his statements with "well, most people need much more support than I do".

I want for everyone what walking affords me. It doesn't need to be the physical. It can be the social, emotional and mental health benefits that are much more impactful anyway. Clearing the way for everyone to have access to this experience is a big job and it's one I take very seriously.

Walkability and walking is key to the future of health. It's easy, free and functional. Getting our families outside, walking through life is good for all of us and good for the environment. If there was one change I would love to make for every Australian, it's to ask all governments, councils, and property developers to keep on prioritising our walkability for future planning and development. It works.

5. Data

I would like to acknowledge the work of Dr Oliver Canfell for his co-authorship of this piece. Oliver is a passionate dietitian and researcher dedicated to preventing and managing obesity across the life course. Oliver has been active in obesity research and practice in Queensland, Australia at a clinical, community, and public health level, and is forever proud of being part of Queensland's leadership in this area. He is a previous PhD student of mine and one of the kindest people on the planet.

Oliver (20-something): I use data to make decisions almost every hour of every day. I plan my public transport route to work with multiple GPS options to figure out the fastest way (the Chief Executive would be pleased). During my supermarket shop at the end of the day, I assess my food budget for the week and admit that I can't afford lettuce or many leafy greens, so I alter my plans and choose canned legumes or cabbage instead.

Rob (40-something): I use data consistently, but I wasn't quite as aware of it until recently. I go for a run, only to be told that I am going at a slow pace today. My phone has told me I have four missed calls and I am about to be late for my first meeting. I receive a reminder from my doctor for my appointment tomorrow, which I use to update my online calendar. I make it to my meeting, try to run a bit faster (only lasting for about 100m) and my doctor was late anyway! This is all through the nudging of my personal data. When did I become so reliant on data?

The era of COVID-19 – and digital transformation.

No matter our age, we make the most informed decisions when data is at our fingertips. This is true on a personal and global level. We have seen the extraordinary value of data as a first-line digital defence against COVID-19. Data underpinned digital surveillance for early COVID-19 detection, new visualisation tools that supported nationwide policy decisions and prediction modelling that informed health system planning for each wave. For the average Australian, it may have been reporting symptoms and helping with contact tracing. This rapid, global digital transformation ushered in a new horizon of 'digital public health'. In its first true test, digital public health helped enormously to manage COVID-19 – a communicable (infectious) disease – but what about digital public health for noncommunicable (chronic) disease? How can a prevention agency – with a remit of good public health policy, starting with obesity prevention – shift towards digital public health to improve Queenslanders' health and wellbeing?

Data is just one piece of the puzzle.

To be clear, decision-making is not – and should certainly not be – a one-piece puzzle, where data is the hero. Data is often our corner pieces, grounding the puzzle and providing much-needed direction. As the middle starts to take shape, there is a healthy, and necessary, blend of other puzzle pieces: community voices and lived experience, equity, innovation, professional experience, strategy and traditional research evidence. The role of data is to complement, not dominate, decision-making. Choosing cabbage instead of lettuce might be innovative for Oliver, but based on experience, he knows a coleslaw can be just as delicious as a Caesar salad.

The best decisions for prevention and the best decisions for us, are those that are led by us. Decisions need every piece of the puzzle, with data as a cornerstone. In our opinion, there are several reasons that make data critical to the success of prevention:

Data is a powerful storytelling tool.

The true power of data lies in its ability to tell a story. The ability to process, remember and communicate stories is something that connects every culture throughout history. Data is not just numbers and modelling; it's yarning, stories, voices, and lived experience. Data-driven storytelling helps us to understand our environment, so we can push back as we see it influencing us. Data helps us by providing clarity on what's happening. You can look at the graphs your bank and electricity providers send you, to understand the story of your usage. This helps you decide whether you are going to use the washing line (instead of the dryer) and reminds you to turn the air conditioners off more frequently.

Where to from here?

Oliver (20-something): As a researcher and health professional, I am not afraid to admit that the power of data excites me. I believe unleashing data in the right ways – responsibly and with precision – will mean a healthier future generation of Queenslanders. The more we embrace data and digital as an agent for more efficient, prevention-driven healthcare, the greater our impact on reducing chronic diseases will be.

Rob (40-something): As a leader in the health system, I want to ensure we make a difference in a complicated world. The future is big, complex and different. We need all types of information to help us make an informed decision. Data is critical to help guide us in making the big decisions at a population level, just as it is part of our decision-making when choosing which doctor to use or how best to set reminders for meetings. The more I know about data, the less it scares me. Data alone will not make the decision but will help us to make the most informed ones.

Again, it's about understanding our environment and arming ourselves with the information to influence back.

6. **Climate change**
   I would like to acknowledge Emeritus Professor Ian Lowe, Griffith University and Health and Wellbeing Queensland Board member, who is a true expert in Australia, for writing this with me. Recently recognised as one of the top 100 Australian Scientists, highlights his exceptional contributions to environmental science, urban development, sustainability,

and public health. I am so privileged to work with leaders of this calibre.

Throughout Australia, we have had a multitude of challenges to contend with. COVID-19, bushfires and floods have truly had an impact on the lives of our population, especially those most vulnerable. Our physical health and our mental health have suffered. For some of us, our financial security has deteriorated and we now find it even more difficult to put food on the table for our loved ones. 2024 is no different.

The health of all Australians goes hand in hand with planetary health

When we think of climate change, most of us think about the increasing frequency and intensity of extreme weather events such as heat waves, bushfires, floods, droughts and storms. It still seems hard to make the connection between this and poor health. However, did you know that climate change does not just mean an increase in average temperature year after year? It has dramatically increased the number of very hot days that we experience. One figure demonstrates this perfectly. From 1900 to 1980, in an average year there were three or four days that were the hottest in our recorded history. In 2020, a remarkable 43 days were the hottest ever recorded. Heat waves are a direct threat to human health.

With hot weather, vegetation gets drier and the risk of severe bushfires increases. The fires of the 2019-20 summer were unprecedented. A hotter world means more water goes into the atmosphere, resulting in more intense rainfall events like the so-called 'rain bomb' that hit south-east Queensland and northern New South Wales earlier this year. These events destroy huge areas of natural vegetation, thousands of homes and significant public infrastructure, resulting in a loss of human lives.

The damage (physical, financial and mental health impact) doesn't repair itself overnight. The effects of such devastating events can be long-lasting and life-altering. Unpredictable climate is causing distress and mental health issues, particularly for Queenslanders in rural areas. As rural production struggles, so do the towns that depend on the farming sector. 'Eco-anxiety' is emerging for children and young people as they struggle with foreseeable deterioration of our planet. Educators reported that their students commonly experienced feeling overwhelmed, hopeless, anxious, angry, sad and frustrated when engaging with ecological crises.

Healthy people are needed to maintain a healthy planet
Helping people to be healthy can have positive environmental outcomes. This can help reduce the health care sector's environmental footprint by decreasing carbon emissions, waste production, water and energy usage, and inefficient models of care. Prioritising preventive health can keep people out of the health system.

Current efforts in public health
According to the world's leading medical journal, *The Lancet*, global efforts to tackle climate change represent one of the greatest opportunities to improve public health this century. At Health and

Wellbeing Queensland, we are working together to understand the link between climate change and health, ultimately supporting the work needed to protect our health as we learn how. It's simply the best thing we can do to improve the life expectancy of our next generation, to ensure our children live the longest and healthiest lives they are entitled to.

Our food system
Right now, recent climate events are impacting the security of our food and the availability and price of healthy food. In Queensland, the McKell Institute's Food Insecurity Index shows Central and North Queensland have a food insecurity score 60 per cent higher than inner Brisbane. We are working with remote and First Nations communities to support local sustainable food production, access to healthy food and healthy homes, so households can choose, prepare, cook and store healthy food options at all times. This also results in less transportation of food, which reduces the carbon footprint across the supply chain.

Working locally, and strengthening farmer and food connections, is important as food security directly effects the health of the diets we provide for our families.

Our diets play a role in climate change. Healthy diets have an appropriate energy intake and consist of a diversity of plant-based foods, low amounts of animal source foods, unsaturated rather than saturated fats and prioritises wholegrains with minimal refined grains. We need these foods to be available and accessible to our communities right across the country. Our job is not only to support agriculture to produce such healthy food, but also to ensure it is accessible and affordable, no matter where they live.

Our physical activity system

Using petroleum fuels for urban transport directly causes local air pollution which causes a range of respiratory diseases. This is where Brisbane should be congratulated on public transport. Brisbane City Council decided more than 20 years ago to phase out diesel buses and replace them with gas-powered vehicles, a policy which has contributed to significantly cleaner air.

But many people commute by car in our towns and cities, a practice which is both causing worse air pollution and directly causing injuries from road accidents, a problem that is so predictable we call it 'the road toll'.

Lack of physical activity is also a contributor to people living with overweight or obesity. Those who walk or cycle to work, study or shops, obviously get more exercise, but so do those who use public transport, which requires walking to and from the journey end-points. So, we need to think not just about transport choices, but also about the urban planning decisions that determine whether the services people use regularly are within walking or cycling distance, or at least accessible by reliable and safe public transport.

The public health opportunity is now

Climate change affects our health, and what people do affects the health of our planet. The most exciting part about this story is that we can make a difference and drive real change, more than ever before. When we include thinking about planetary health, the co-benefits are immense: health (such as better nutrition and reduced obesity rates), economic (people can be more physically active with an environment that supports them to do so) and environmental (helping our farmers to navigate the challenges the current weather and climate is throwing at them).

Climate change may seem like an odd topic to include in a book about your health and wellbeing, but there is a direct link and it's really important we talk about it. If our planet isn't healthy, it becomes very difficult for us to be healthy. Take extreme heat, for example. Climate change has increased the number of hot days we experience, and this extreme heat directly affects our health and wellbeing. More hot days increases the risk of bushfires (because of dry vegetation) and severe rain events (as more water goes into the atmosphere). These weather events destroy vegetation, property, livelihoods and often result in loss of human life. The financial, physical and mental health impacts are huge. Recovery is long, if at all. People's lives change forever. And for those not directly involved, the flow on effect often means shortages and price increases for healthy foods. You might remember the price of lettuce skyrocketing to more than $10 for a single lettuce after severe flooding in parts of the country. The availability and cost of fresh fruits and vegetables is directly affected by weather events!

Our children are also feeling the effects of climate change. I am told that many of our children worry about what is happening to our planet and are experiencing what has been termed 'eco-anxiety'. Our children shouldn't have to worry about this.

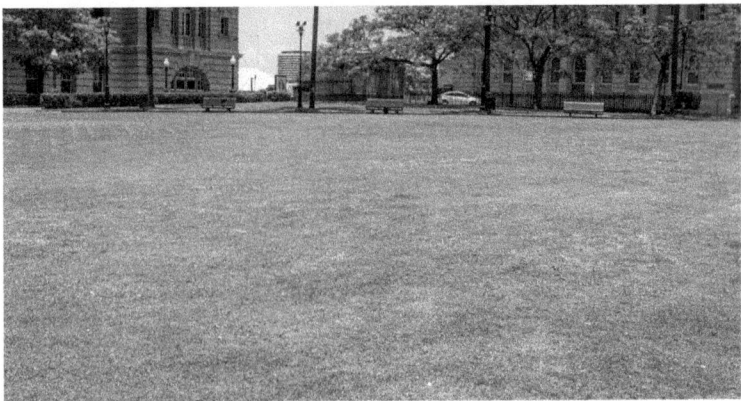

In 2024, there is a lot of work underway by governments and organisations to reduce our carbon footprint and to improve the health of our planet. Strategies that make it easier for people to drive less and exercise more are good for the environment and our health. While strategies to support local sustainable food production will mean families have access to food at all times, they also reduce the need for food transportation (reducing the carbon footprint). It is truly a systems solution we need. We must think broadly and long term.

7. **Women**

We need truly transformative change to dismantle the strong barriers holding gender imbalance in place. We need to be different, be bold and most importantly, be together. For me, change of that significance is always generational. Bold, big, progressive change is most successful when perspectives and expectations shift towards the next generation rather than their own. It always means solutions are much more sustainable.

In my own life, gender equity is never far from my mind and in fact, is relevant in every role I hold. It often consumes my thinking… but not for myself. I am talking about gender equity for our kids, our young girls and boys and how we have to ensure mindsets, policies and practices that shift towards supporting gender equity are also consuming young minds, in a very positive way.

I am disappointed to say that I still see examples where the focus is skewed towards disrespecting men, to try to drive an equitable playing field for women. In my mind, there has never been any cause for disrespect of the male gender. This is not fair and most importantly, it doesn't get us anywhere.

Put simply, I have three beautiful sons. They have done nothing wrong. Why would I ever suggest that, because of their gender, the gender gap is widening? It's simply not true.

My thinking is just so different and always has been. It has always informed how I live my life. I wanted to explain that. I have five ways and five lessons I have learned on how to do this – big, bold and differently for real change, my way.

1. Role model how you want to be treated, the respect you want to receive and how you want the world to be. Your children are watching every single thing you do.
2. Give back if you are in leadership roles. Afford to others what you have been afforded (and make deliberate and conscious efforts to do this).
3. Influence social media in a very positive way. Be deliberate here too. It is possible.
4. Invest your time and/or resources (whatever you have control over) to drive an agenda that will empower women and girls whenever you are able to.
5. Ensure women understand the environment around them and the factors promoting those barriers in place.

Although gender is one of the most significant social determinants of health outcomes, the global health community is largely unaware of the different circumstances and outcomes experienced between different genders. The biological differences in men and women do not fully explain the worldwide differences in health outcomes observed throughout history and across the globe. The current women are more likely to have two or more chronic conditions compared to males *(21% and 16% respectively),* with a higher prevalence of mental or behavioural conditions, anxiety, osteoporosis and chronic obstructive pulmonary disease among women.

Of this entire section, focus on respect for all. The next generation of Queenslanders are good, kind and respectful. They should never be made to feel that their gender is to blame for previous inequities. Enlist them to drive a strong agenda to close the gender gap with you. My boys are crystal clear on how they empower women. They just have to do more of the same throughout their lives. If that happens, my job here is done.

8. Parenting

I am privileged to be the mother of three beautiful boys; now young men. My children have been relentlessly supported by a full-time working mother throughout their lives, from the minute they were born until the present day. They are respectful of both women and men, and I am yet to see a single occurrence where their values regarding gender have been compromised. They are equally respectful, sensitive, understanding and supportive of both genders. There have been times when I have had to ensure I was not overcompensating to ensure the boys understood this. Examples of this include when my primary school aged twins asked me; Twin one "Mummy, can men be doctors too?" and twin two "Mummy, daddy has gone out. Who will make us dinner?". So, instead of ensuring my boys understood Mummies didn't always have to cook and stay at home to be the carer, equally, I had to ensure they understood, neither did Daddies...

Don't underestimate what your children learn from you by osmosis every single day. It is powerful, use it wisely. They grow up so quickly!

As children grow, they absorb subtle and overt messages about what is valued, who has power and how to behave. Gender socialisation begins at home. However, it is confirmed or reiterated by other influencers/leaders in a children's life including teachers, faith leaders, peers, coaches, siblings and exposure to social media with the latter becoming so much more dominant. By the age of ten, children have already absorbed restrictive norms about acceptable gendered conduct. Research has shown that exposure to counter-stereotypical gender roles alters how an individual forms impressions and processes social information, allowing them to be more individualistic and creative in their thinking - not just in relation to gender roles, but more broadly in life. In other words, children can create their own opinions based on what makes sense to them. I have no doubt this has been the case in my own household. I love that I have given that to my children.

9. Leadership

I have the ultimate privilege of having a voice in Queensland, through government, communities, families and most importantly, young women and girls. The importance of that is never lost on me. This privilege has shaped how I act, what I say, the effort I invest and how deeply I get involved in activities that promote women's empowerment, in the hope to lead change for gender balance: or even thinking that it's possible and I truly believe it is. I reflect on my own career as I worked up through the professional ranks. I did this through hard work and discipline, lots of study and always with the support of other professional women and men who held positions far more senior than I. They empowered me to understand it is possible and that encouragement positioned me well. I'm incredibly grateful for that support and acknowledge that many of them still support me to this day, relentlessly. I consciously pass this on and as a female Chief Executive in Government, I believe it's my privilege, my responsibility and my job, to ensure I do this every day. Mentoring the next generation of Queensland female leaders remains a priority to me, as it was for my mentors. Those informal networks, corridor chats, texts of encouragement, mentoring coffees and phone calls (at just the right time) can often be more powerful than any formal arrangement.

In fact, research suggests that subtle exposure to highly successful female leaders can inspire women's behaviour and self-evaluations in stressful leadership tasks. Every touch point for me with young women is critical, and should be for every woman in a leadership role. In turn, they give so much back to me, as I learn so much about our exciting next generation of Queenslanders.

It is more broadly known that women continue to be underrepresented in leadership roles. Evidence suggests diversity and the inclusion of both women and men in leadership positions is crucial to tackling complex challenges, through the development of innovative and successful approaches. This means a mix of both is needed. Research tells us that addressing the barriers that contribute to the underrepresentation of women in leadership positions today, combined with executive coaching, is important to sustain the next generation of women leaders into the future.

10. Social media

I know what women search for through their social media channels and I know this varies significantly at different times in their lives. In times of success and perceived failure throughout life, we all look for something that will either validate our thinking, make us feel a little better or find help. Like many others, I was that person and I still am. Unfortunately, I'm still very aware of how disempowering some of the imagery and messaging communicated through marketing and social media can be, especially for those women who are faced with more vulnerable circumstances. Just as racism exists, misogyny and discrimination are much more pronounced in social media forums. So-called 'keyboard warriors' are both cowardly and dangerous in equal measure. While many choose to respond with sarcasm or vitriol, I also see an opportunity to re-present the facts and the evidence to someone who is at least engaged in the conversation! Through all of my own personal channels and that of Health and Wellbeing Queensland, my team and I will always take the time to get it right, use the power of positive messaging and empowerment, and this will never change. In fact, I will never respond to negativity and words of oppression.

Through the isolation of COVID-19, we certainly saw social media providing a way for many people, including women, to generate or increase their income, gain awareness of their rights and improve their own and their families' wellbeing. Let's use this growth to our advantage.

We also know that women are more likely to seek health information online than men. A previous study conducted in Australia showed 44 per cent of women aged 18-23 years referred to the internet as a source of health information, with high potential of online resources to address stigmatising and sensitive health issues. Empowering women with credible sources of information will not only promote positive decisions for themselves, but also for their children, helping to improve outcomes for our next generation.

WHAT THIS MEANS FOR YOUR VILLAGE

To understand what these factors are, how they are influencing you and what you can expect, provides you with a defence mechanism for you to influence back. You can get your village ready to manage any impacts that may affect you, your family or your community. With knowledge comes power and with power comes influence. You are in control.

Chapter 5 References

89. Health and Wellbeing Queensland. 2020. *Opinion Articles* [Online]. Brisbane, Queensland, Australia: Queensland Government. Available: https://hw.qld.gov.au/blog/category/opinion/ [Accessed 2023].

90. Lowe, I. 2023. *Why Australia needs to change its thinking on growing the economy* [Online]. Sydney Morning Herald. Available: https://www.smh.com.au/environment/sustainability/why-australia-needs-to-change-its-thinking-on-growing-the-economy-20230404-p5cy04.html [Accessed 2023].

91. Wellbeing Economy Alliance. 2022. *New Zealand - Implementing the Wellbeing Budget* [Online]. Available: https://weall.org/resource/new-zealand-implementing-the-wellbeing-budget [Accessed 2023].

92. Government of New Zealand. 2020. *Wellbeing Budget 2020: Rebuilding Together* [Online]. Government of New Zealand. Available: https://www.treasury.govt.nz/publications/wellbeing-budget/wellbeing-budget-2020#from-the-prime-minister [Accessed 2023].

93. KPMG. 2022. *Shifting the dial on vegetable consumption – Rebuilding healthy families in a COVID-19 affected and disrupted Australia* [Online]. Available: https://static1.squarespace.com/static/5ddca44a3ac7644d-97d9757a/t/633e2e9e396cdd49ccfa3ee9/1665019635620/FVC+Report_Final_041022.pdf [Accessed 2023].

94. Queensland Government. 2019. *Queensland Walking Strategy 2019-2029. Walking: for everyone, every day* [Online]. Transport and Main Roads. Available: https://www.tmr.qld.gov.au/-/media/Travelandtransport/Pedestrians-and-walking/

Queensland-Walking-Strategy-2019-2029.pdf?la=en [Accessed 2023].

95. Olshansky, S. J., Passaro, D. J., Hershow, R. C., Layden, J., Carnes, B. A., Brody, J., Hayflick, L., Butler, R. N., Allison, D. B. & Ludwig, D. S. 2005. A potential decline in life expectancy in the United States in the 21st century. *N Engl J Med,* 352, 1138-45.

96. Australian Institute of Health and Welfare. 2023. *Chronic Disease* [Online]. AIHW. Available: https://www.aihw.gov.au/reports-data/health-conditions-disability-deaths/chronic-disease/overview [Accessed 2023].

97. Australian Institute of Health and Welfare. 2022. *Disease expenditure in Australia 2019-20* [Online]. AIHW. Available: https://www.aihw.gov.au/getmedia/f1a20cd3-c24c-45e4-ae00-9a6f9c95903c/Disease-expenditure-in-Australia-2019-20.pdf.aspx?inline=true [Accessed 2023].

98. Greenhalgh, E., Hurley, S, Lal, A. 2020. *17.4 Economic evaluations of tobacco control interventions* [Online]. Melbourne: Cancer Council Victoria. Available: https://www.tobaccoinaustralia.org.au/chapter-17-economics/17-4-economic-evaluations-of-tobacco-control-interventions [Accessed 2023].

CHAPTER 6

Our legacy

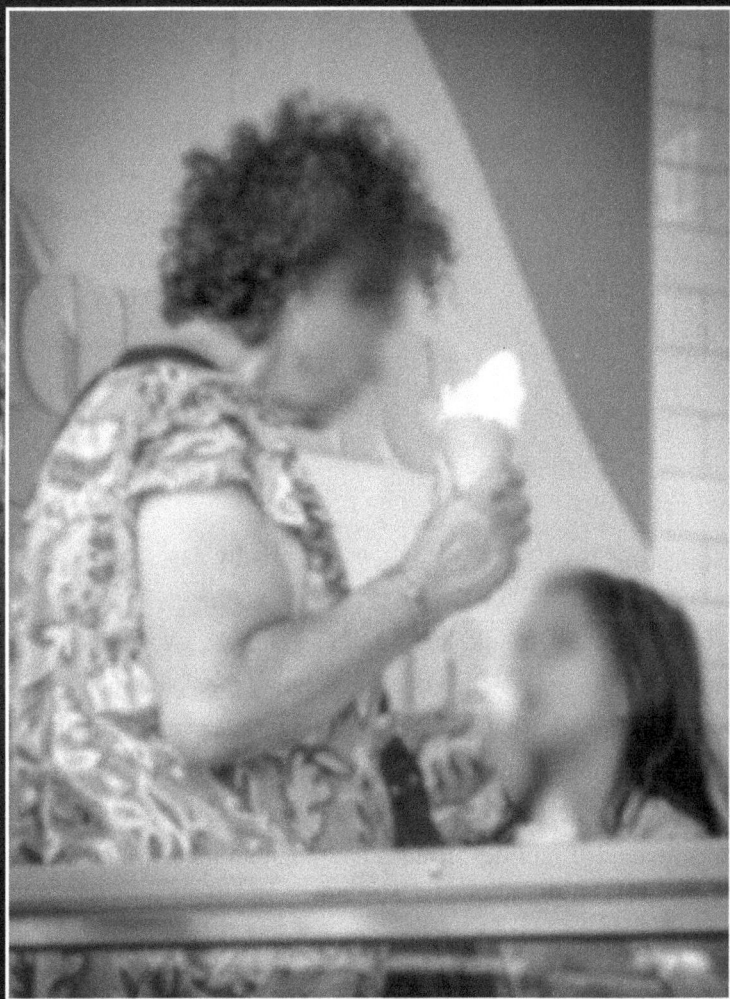

CHAPTER 6

Our legacy

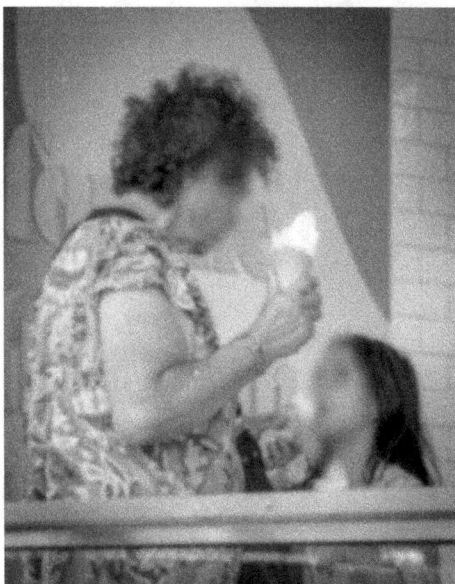

So where are we today?

We need to go 'back to the future'. If you're sick and tired of your parents saying, 'In my day...', you may not want to read on. However, if you're not, then you will love this.

In my day...

Yes, back in the 1970s and 80s we did a good job. We ate better, we moved more, we watched one screen at a time, had much less screen time, and often had to get up to change the channel and flick through our wide variety of three channels and ABC (previously known as Channel 2). We seemed to do a lot more with our parents, extended families, friends and communities. We created 'villages' who would help protect us from the challenges of the social determinants, which stand in the way of progress.

On the weekends, at about 6am, my friends and I packed our backpacks with a vegemite sandwich, a piece of fruit and a frozen water bottle, loaded up our bikes and took off. I would always end up at the local creek, swam, caught yabbies and played in local horse stables where 'visitors would be prosecuted' apparently, we would explore all day. I would climb trees, take the macadamia nuts and custard apples from vacated properties and sell them on the side of the road. Throughout my childhood, I would have completed thousands of kilometres riding around the cul-de-sac on my bike. I would be gone all day and arrive home just as the sun was setting to a hot meal waiting on the table. I had to send my friends home as there was not enough food for more than the four of us. The food was purchased, prepared and dished up as four perfectly portioned parts onto medium size plates. There were no leftovers and no additional sauces, 'jus or caramelised vinaigrettes. We had the choice of water or milk to drink, the dog was fed and placed outside and the television was off and the table was set. We had to wash our hands before sitting down and we would never start eating until we were all seated and ready. Dinner was never rushed.

When you think back, this was a routine, a ceremony, a celebration of our family and of our day. We kept our elbows off the table, took our time and ate until we were full. However, the sheer fact that the whole process required at least 45 minutes of our time, meant our bodies had the luxury to feel full. Messages from our brain could be sent to our body, telling us clearly that if you keep eating, you are going to feel bloated and sick. We would stop eating as a result.

If I was lucky, mum would let me jump on the trampoline for another 20 minutes after dinner with the floodlights on (we didn't have those on very long as they were very expensive to run). As an alternative, we would have a quick swim after dinner, which was always a delightful surprise when Dad suggested it.

When baths were done, we knew we could sit down and watch A Country Practice until 8.30pm and it was my favourite hour of the day. I would sit on the beanbag. The whole family enjoyed this time together too. At the end of the show, my sister and I knew it was bedtime. There was no negotiation. We would wind down in the hour watching A Country Practice, clean our teeth in the ad breaks and bring our lunchboxes to the kitchen to be filled for the next day. The dog would come in and sit on the mat inside the back screen door with us.

I would kiss everyone goodnight and get into bed at 8.30pm (on the dot). The lights were always off but I could leave my door open for some light if I wanted to read; but only for 10-15 minutes if I couldn't sleep. Every night I would peer out the security screened window and could always see the moon. I remember always feeling relaxed and tired when I went to bed.

Children of my era expected to live to the same age or longer than their parents. Sadly, things have changed.

Research published by Health and Wellbeing Queensland in 2022, reported that "Children born in 2023, are likely to have a shorter life than their parents". This is based on data measuring the

Queensland population specifically and is alarmingly following the same trends that were first reported in the United States in the New England Journal of Medicine (2005). Olshansky (a world-famous Professor of Public Health) with his team, reported that life expectancy across America will decrease by one third to three fourths of a year, due to the negative impact of obesity on life expectancy.[95] There was much uproar about this publication and prediction as this was the first time in a developed country that life expectancy was not only predicted to stop increasing, it was actually going to decline. This attracted huge debate, negative response and reaction from the public, as well as experts who accused Professor Olshansky of "playing politics instead of science". Unfortunately, for the population of the United States of America, Olshansky's predictions were wrong. In fact, the decline came much faster than he predicted.

Released on 2 November 2022, the Queensland State Government released data predicting a decline in life expectancy for the Queensland population by up to 4.1 years and up to 5 years for our precious First Nations communities. In addition to this, we know that one in two Australian adults (47%) were living with one or more chronic conditions in 2020-21,[96] costing the Australian health care system $140.4 billion in 2019-20.[97]
So, what do we do?

This article suggests we go back to the conditions of the 1980s. I agree entirely. However, I want to break this down to be clear.

In Australia, there has been so much progress in certain areas through strong public health effort. Specifically in Queensland, the Governor of Queensland, Her Excellency the Honourable Dr Jeannette Young AC PSM, the former Queensland Chief Health Officer, drove a relentless, strong and relevant policy to ban smoking. Defending much push back and debate, Queensland continued to lead the way in Australia to ban smoking and as a result, smoking control interventions are estimated to have saved the Australian economy $8.06 billion through a reduction in disease rates and premature deaths.[98] This was a huge milestone for Australia, and I continue to celebrate our very own Queensland Governor for making such a difference.

Smoking rates should continue to decline, smoking bans should continue to increase and vaping should now be targeted as a major increasing risk and public health issue. We can learn from this.

However, just from my very simplistic life story above, the other social conditions or determinants could and should reflect more closely the conditions experienced 40 years ago. They could include:

1. Eating – the way we eat, what we purchase, take-aways, where we eat in the house, the ceremony of meals, simplicity of meals, portion sizes, fruit and vegetables on every plate, the way we shop and how we dish up meals on plates needs to make a comeback. Can we achieve thriving gardens (either in our own backyard or collective areas within communities) where we can grow tomatoes, beans or even honeysuckles (and suck the honey out of the flowers)? Does anyone even know what that means today?

2. Screen time – screen time (aka television) should be negotiated, limited and used in different ways. No screens should be allowed in bedrooms, as this will only increase and escalate anxiety and keep you awake or wake you during the night. Can we go to sleep without the need for deep sound waves, ocean life or Frasier-repeats on the iPad?

3. Sleep routine – go to bed at the same time and wake up at the same time. Know when bedtime is and make sure you, your children and entire family have some time to 'wind down' before you actually get into bed. Lights must go off as darkness will only support you to achieve deep sleep for longer.

4. Play – to be clear, I'm not saying to go out all day, play in prohibited areas and return in the dark. However, there needs to be a time and place for all of us (children and adults) to feel free to move around, explore and refresh. Scheduled play and sports times are good, however, flexible play, unmapped walks and enjoyment in the environment is so good for your health.

5. Physical activity – to me, this is about allowing our kids to be kids again. Can our kids safely walk to school? Can our kids play in the playground before the school bell without being told to sit down as the 'handball game' is too risky? Can we have better use of school grounds outside school hours – using the ovals as dog parks, picnic areas or

unscheduled areas of free play (backyard cricket) – and whatever happened to totem tennis?

6. Drinks – can we really 'just drink water?'. Again, for clarity, I am not suggesting you don't drink any milk or dairy. However, for our main drink, I am suggesting water is the best chance we've got to maintain as a lifelong habit. Water at the dinner table, water in our water bottles and glasses on our desk at work and clean water for all communities across the entire state is what I'm suggesting. Whoever introduced sports drinks, soft drinks and cordials to market to children, non-athletes and communities experiencing vulnerability have a lot to answer for. Just ... Drink ... Water, just as we used to. It will do us the world of good.

7. Mental wellbeing - I have kept the most important for last. I have always experienced very good mental wellbeing. I actually had all the elements of it, grew it, supported it and nurtured my wellbeing, without even knowing it. To me, that's the beauty of going back from the future. We simply didn't know we were being healthy, it was just the way we lived, and our wellbeing excelled as a result. I had time to play, I had freedom to explore, and spent time outside, got caught in the rain at times and was never rushed. The full exposure and impact of dangerous marketing never impacted me and purchasing a 600ml Coke buddy or upsized McDonald's meal deals weren't even a thing. I was comfortable with my routine. I was

aware of my screen time limits aka A Country Practice, I knew my bedtime and wake up routine. I didn't have the pressure of worrying about my diet, my weight, my step count or my sleep cycles. I didn't care whether my balsamic was caramelised and I slept well. I wasn't shamed by celebrity bodies, I wasn't bullied on social media and didn't care about the numbers of friends or 'likes' I had. My mealtimes were good. I knew I could talk to my family about any problems, or they could see when something was bothering me. We had face-to-face time every day. Today, that's a luxury.

In my life today, I follow all these factors above. It doesn't cost me more and my mental health is strong. I don't feel guilty or anxious if I don't get to the gym or do a scheduled run. However, I am changing the environment around me to support my community, my family and my life. This is all I want for you... but I will help you.

My job as Queensland's leader in Prevention is to support you, not blame you. It is to ensure I understand what works, what doesn't and how I can best make you aware of all of it.

What I am describing here is changes in the environment. It's not changes to your personal responsibility. If you take nothing else out away from this book, please take this:

The environment has changed. Life is faster today, people have more chronic diseases, we are consuming more convenient, faster food; moving less and doing much more using screens. We are sleeping less; keeping our phones on during the night next to our bed and making no time for our own wellbeing. We feel worse about ourselves and remain unmotivated, alongside feeling terrible about that too. It is a vicious cycle that we simply must stop.

People have continued to do as they are being told. Labels such as "healthy, light, low fat, healthy choice and lite" are being applied flippantly but not accidentally. Health star ratings don't always mean what you think they do and there may be a food cue (reminding us to eat) every 50 metres.

Where you live makes such a difference. Communities experiencing greater vulnerability with higher chronic disease rates, are targeted by fast-food and other private industries. In fact, financially, some of us have no choice but to buy high fat, take-aways to feed their families with the cost of living increasing.

My point here is that for many of us, there is no choice. The environment has worked against us, as many of us have done what we have been 'steered' towards.

Once you know that, life will become easier. Take the pressure off yourself. There is no blame and there should be no guilt for anything you feel you are not getting right.

WHAT THIS MEANS FOR YOUR VILLAGE:
Let's start with understanding the words in this book. I am clearly saying if you live in Australia, you have the right to good health.

Going back to basics, embracing some of your or your parents social conditions growing up, can help.

Start with the top seven above.

Ease into it. Don't be so hard on yourself.

This change will mean something different to everyone, as we all don't start from the same place. After all, our lives cannot be about chance. It can be about change and it might be time for you to do it. Personally, I will continue to lead the change to the environment to support the top seven.

You and I together can create a brilliant village for our children. It's actually the way it used to work and it's right.

Chapter 6 References

1. Olshansky, S. J., Passaro, D. J., Hershow, R. C., Layden, J., Carnes, B. A., Brody, J., Hayflick, L., Butler, R. N., Allison, D. B. & Ludwig, D. S. 2005. A potential decline in life expectancy in the United States in the 21st century. *N Engl J Med,* 352, 1138-45.

2. Australian Institute of Health and Welfare. 2023. *Chronic Disease* [Online]. AIHW. Available: https://www.aihw.gov.au/reports-data/health-conditions-disability-deaths/chronic-disease/overview [Accessed 2023].

3. Australian Institute of Health and Welfare. 2022. *Disease expenditure in Australia 2019-20* [Online]. AIHW. Available: https://www.aihw.gov.au/getmedia/f1a20cd3-c24c-45e4-ae00-9a6f9c95903c/Disease-expenditure-in-Australia-2019-20.pdf.aspx?inline=true [Accessed 2023].

4. Greenhalgh, E., Hurley, S, Lal, A. 2020. *17.4 Economic evaluations of tobacco control interventions* [Online]. Melbourne: Cancer Council Victoria. Available: https://www.tobaccoinaustralia.org.au/chapter-17-economics/17-4-economic-evaluations-of-tobacco-control-interventions [Accessed 2023].

Where can I go to find help?

I am conscious that most books today back up their work with a website and send their readers to it to find a range of tools, information and fact sheets, to all people to implement the changes they have made more easily. This is often very useful, especially for books referring people looking for mental wellbeing and psychological support. I am not going to do that as I don't think it will help the current population by giving yet another option to consider when looking for good nutrition information. In my professional opinion as a Dietitian, one thing I am absolutely sure of is, there is too much duplication of information, too much inconsistent information, too much misinformation and too much wrong information. The nutrition and wellbeing environment is a full and busy one, and extremely hard to navigate (even as an expert). How do you possibly separate fact from fiction?

You don't have to. I want to direct you to the only place where Dietitians, Exercise Physiologists, Paediatricians, Endocrinologists, General Practitioners, Nurses, Teachers, Lawyers and other health professionals have come together to write the information, recommend further reading and support, where there are multiple options to choose from when considering improving your wellbeing and where all resources are absolutely free of charge. Further, these resources were never available when I was growing up in my family (and local community), starting out as a health professional and as a mother, raising my children. I want to ensure everyone takes full advantage of what the four Health Promotion Agencies across Australia provide. The work is credible, evidence-based, innovative and independent. That means you don't need to put so much effort into the integrity of the work. They have done it all for you. They are actual gifts afforded to all Australians and sadly, most of us don't even know they exist. Please visit the websites below. I am not sure I have seen anything better anywhere in the world:

For Queensland, I want to refer you to Health and Wellbeing Queensland.

Health and Wellbeing Queensland Website

Health and Wellbeing Queensland Instagram Page

Health and Wellbeing Queensland Facebook Page

Whether you want cooking advice and recipes, access to walking programs, free coaching sessions or information on raising children (and safe introduction to solids), this is an excellent resource and starting point.

VicHealth is equally brilliant. Preventative Health SA and Healthway (WA) are also outstanding for finding information, funding opportunities and functional, credible support.

Health promotion and wellbeing organisations/agencies are the way of the future and I encourage you to get to know what's available to you. I wish someone had told me about them years ago.

Looking toward 2025 and beyond

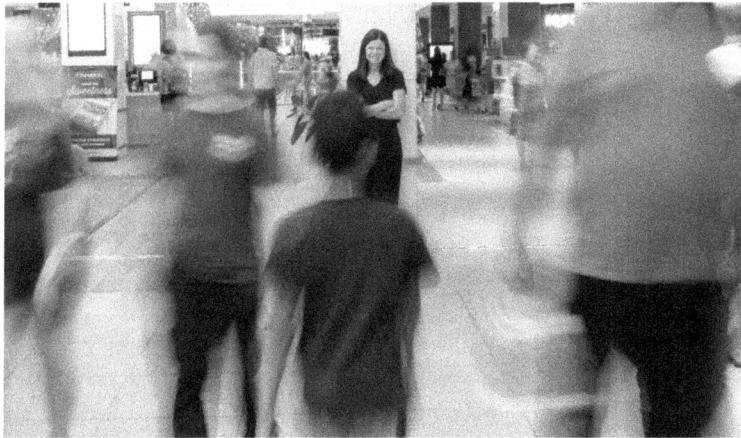

2024 has already declared itself. I feel things are more definite, impactful and all encompassing. For me, this is not a year for outrageous celebrations and events. This is a year for hard work, recovery, peace, kindness and building back up our own health and wellbeing and to help those around us to build theirs. It's a time to look inwards, both personally and strengthen your own little villages – your family village, your work village, your town and your friendship villages and see what your village needs or what more you can do.

Overwhelmed by weather events globally, the first months of 2024 in Australia have been difficult, although not unexpected or unpredicted. Rain, cyclones, flooding and tornados have dominated the news and our lives, ensuring a quick transition from Christmas celebrations to saving lives from natural disasters.

For me personally, the beginning of 2024 has been even tougher. The decline of my Father's health has meant alongside my mother and sister, I have adjusted my life to care for him through problem-solving, pivoting and doing what I can to make the end of his life better. Doing this has brought so much joy to all of us. Spending time with my Dad throughout this period has been both emotional and yet reaffirming that our village makes such a difference.

Dad has always created supportive villages in all aspects of his life. During his working life, the success of his organisation and his usual 80 hour working weeks were highly dependent on the respect, loyalty and competence of his hard-working staff (some working for Dad for 46 years). Throughout this time, they did their jobs exceptionally well as evidenced by the gifts some of his customers had to pay with (potatoes, cakes, beef) – in today's terms, equivalent to a 5-star Google rating. His staff managed significant logistics in operating several business premises at the peak of the engineering business success, all whilst the business recovered from two significant floods, major theft and vandalism. Dad needed a work village that was amazing and led by him, they never let him down. In my opinion, he created a workplace spanning 50 years where people wanted to work, a big industry and most importantly, truck drivers from around Australia knew they had a friend whenever they had a problem. Dad's village was big, exciting and all-encompassing but also respectful, happy and loving. Despite the enormity of his work, Dad was grounded and very well liked. He was most grateful for his home-made lunches, his freezing cold water taps (which was quite innovative many decades ago), his crisp, starched and ironed overalls, his well ironed underpants, handkerchief and long socks. He always smelled clean and he always wore his branding which he was so famous for (Fortuna Engineering), which still stands today proudly in Coopers Plains, Brisbane. This was my Dad's work village for half a century.

In hospital, Dad's village today varies in magnitude, but not in what matters. The health professional workforce supporting Dad's treatment remains respectful, patient and have told me 'they love being around him'. For him right now, his village continues to be made up of respect. He is in hospital and long term care. Even when struggling to breathe with oxygen support, my Father would introduce me, my mother and sister, to the health team every time they entered the room. He loved the smell of the alcohol wipes and I would clean his bedside table every day with them. I would buy a cold water daily and purchased a $19 fan from Kmart that he could control himself. I bought a string of fairy lights that hung above his bed and he ensured the batteries were replaced as often as required and they still hang above his head today. They were very well maintained. A Health and Wellbeing Queensland cap remains on his head. The branding, the crisp clean smell, the respect for everyone in the room and his fairy lights somehow brought meaning to Dad's last little village he created (the fairy lights just brought joy and purpose). His environment, his village, is keeping him happy and comfortable. For me personally, the future is all about the excitement of opportunity to build better health and wellbeing, especially for those who need it the most. Amidst these truly unsettling times, within current community safety challenges, cost of living crisis and housing issues, love and respect for others and the desire to re-create our supportive villages hasn't dissipated. It's simply lying dormant as some of the other negative barriers have taken hold (gaining some traction through the pandemic). Reminding communities of the value of redeveloping their own villages is key and will be enough to start the rebuild. We all have a job to do here.

Our environments also have a role to play, and we need to also hold them to account. Starting with embracing prevention of chronic diseases before requiring treatment is critical. With one in two people in Australia now living with one or more chronic diseases, this should be a major driver to continue to change. Prevention should be much more of a priority for all countries. The concept of the wellbeing economy also needs another look. This sends a clear message that money isn't everything and putting the health and wellbeing of our people first is priority. This new world would support the opportunity of cities hosting global events such as the Olympic and Paralympic Games differently, to remain firmly focussed on the long-term benefits of a strong health legacy for people and our planet, rendering the conversation of structures and 'things' as secondary only. In other words, start the conversation with how we position global investment to support the health of generations to come, using sport, nutrition, wellbeing, and any other opportunities that should and can be leveraged to achieve that as we clean up our environment. It's not the costs and expenditure we have to look hard at, it's the investment.

Building villages at every level is my goal and my pledge to the next generation of Queenslanders. For the health of my children and my children's children.

ObeCity – but not for much longer.

Acknowledgements

There have been decades in the making of this book with the recognition firmly sitting with the children and families I have worked with over the years (as per my introduction). In addition, I would like to thank two people who have committed to getting this work to progress to publication. They have worked both patiently and passionately to make sure I was able to share my learnings through these words. A very big thankyou to Rebecca Griffin, Founder, The PR Firm, who approached me from the very start to write from my own experiences, and to Jessica Hardt, Dietitian and PhD Scholar, who understands how important this work is and has contributed to both the factual information, data and references to ensure we have been accurate and current in all of our storytelling. This book would not be in existence without the two of you. I will miss the group emails with the subject 'That Book'.

In 2024, Professor Ian Lowe was recognised as one of the top 100 scientists in Australia. He is an authority on climate issues and an expert in health and wellbeing. His addition to this book – writing the Foreword - makes a difference. It is yet another example of someone who continues to create villages for people, organisations and communities, determined to leave this world in a better place for our children. Most recently, Professor Lowe has cleared the way for us to improve the health and wellbeing for Queenslanders and I have multiple examples of his impact. His Foreword is extraordinary and something my village is eternally grateful for.

I would also like to recognise the work of Her Excellency the Honourable Dr Jeannette Young AC PSM, Governor of Queensland, who started this strong prevention agenda, led the work and carved this out as a priority for the state of Queensland. We all stand on the shoulders of giants and I am clear Her Excellency, Dr Young, is one of those giants in prevention. I thank her for trusting me to continue to drive this agenda into the future as I take the responsibility very seriously.

To my own 'Littlewood Village'. Whether you are a part of my home village, work village, pilates, academic, walking, friendship, education or any other village we have created together, thank you for living the values alongside me. They are not negotiable and remain unconditional. You have taught me that and I remain a happy and empowered leader in Queensland because of you.

My new 'book village' created this book. In fact, many of my friends and family helped me put this book together. This group of lovely, supportive and committed individuals with very similar values have established our own 'book village' and this is what has compelled me to progress with this project. Without my 'book village', ObeCITY would never have happened.

I want to recognise the work of Health and Wellbeing Queensland. As a brand-new public health agency in Queensland, it has a very big job which is to improve the health of the next generation of Queenslanders. Although I have written this book independently of the organisation, it is the bold and progressive nature of our work that inspires me to do more, such as publish my first manuscript. Thank you to the Health and Wellbeing Queensland Board and Executive team for allowing me to use the blogs we have developed together and for the incredible work you do on a daily basis. Every part of this work gives me hope and I am grateful in Queensland that I have access to something as brilliant as this.

Finally, this book was never written to make money. In fact, the purpose was to empower those who needed it the most. With this as priority, I will ensure any proceeds from this book will be distributed to Not-For-Profit organisations who drive an empowerment, wellbeing and equity agenda, for those who need it.

Everyone in this country has the right to good health. I only hope, either by reading the book or receiving some of the benefits it may create, we will inch a little closer to reaching this goal. It shouldn't be this hard in a beautiful country like Australia.

About the Author

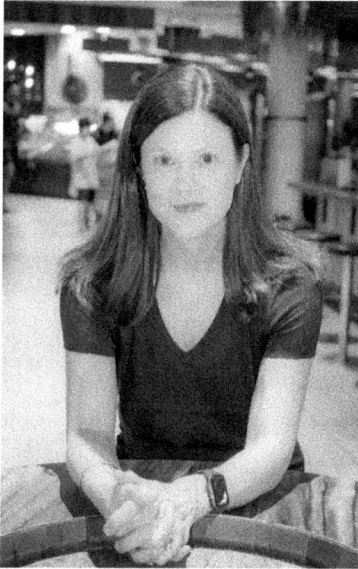

Dr Robyn Littlewood is a very experienced dietitian, educator, professor and senior industry and government leader with more than 25 years' experience working alongside people of all ages, including the most sick and vulnerable children and their families at often the worst times in their lives. Robyn has also advised on nutrition policy in some of the poorest countries and regions globally.

Robyn believes that everyone has the right to good health, no matter who they are or where they live. In this beautiful country of Australia, we should never accept that many of our most precious population, our children, do not have enough to eat, are concerned about the future and often too accepting of poor outcomes and challenges within the environment.

They should expect more, and we should be delivering exactly that. More importantly, everyone should understand their environment, what's working for them and against them. There are deliberate factors that are trying to keep us sick. We can and will do something about it.

As the first Chief Executive Officer of Health and Wellbeing Queensland, Queensland's first prevention agency, Robyn is focused on driving an agenda of fairness and empowerment to ensure the next generation of Queenslanders live healthy and active lives working through all the social factors and determinants that effect health the most.

An experienced leader, researcher, clinician, academic and educator, Robyn holds a raft of formal qualifications in dietetics, business, research and executive leadership from Queensland University of Technology (QUT), James Cook University and The University of Queensland (UQ). These include a PhD, Master of Business Administration, Master of Medical Science and Graduate of the Australian Institute of Company Directors, as well as a Bachelor of Science and formal qualifications in Nutrition and Dietetics.

Before her Chief Executive appointment in 2019, Robyn was a member of the inaugural Health and Wellbeing Queensland Board and held titles including Director, Health Services Research, Children's Health Queensland Hospital and Health Service and Conjoint Associate Professor, Nutrition Science at The University of Queensland. While Director of specialist private nutrition practice ChildD, she led the first national paediatric dietetics training course in Australia, alongside Dietitians Australia, still operating today.

She has also held several Board roles including Board Director,

Dietitians Australia, and has been awarded Fellow, Dietitians Australia for her service. In 2020, Robyn was proudly awarded the Health Alumni of the Year, QUT and the Dietitians Australia, Barbara Chester Award, 2023.

Robyn holds a range of national and Queensland clinical and academic positions and has been an invited speaker at state, national and international conferences. She has produced more than 100 publications, all in the area of children and impacts on health.

Robyn believes every child and family has the right to good health and she is relentless at making sure that happens.

References

2022. National Health Survey. *In:* STATISTICS, A. B. O. (ed.).

2023. Easy Diet Diary. Commercial Banana Bread (regular Slice).

ALLIANCE, W. E. 2022. *New Zealand - Implementing the Wellbeing Budget* [Online]. Available: https://weall.org/resource/new-zealand-implementing-the-wellbeing-budget [Accessed 2023].

ASSOCIATION, A. P. 2023. *Intergenerational trauma* [Online]. Available: https://dictionary.apa.org/intergenerational-trauma [Accessed 2023].

ATTAYE, I., VAN OPPENRAAIJ, S., WARMBRUNN, M. V. & NIEUWDORP, M. 2022. The Role of the Gut Microbiota on the Beneficial Effects of Ketogenic Diets. *Nutrients* [Online], 14.

AUSTRALIA, F. 2023. *Coconut Bread Calories* [Online]. Available: https://www.fatsecret.com.au/calories-nutrition/search?q=Coconut+Bread [Accessed 2023].

AUSTRALIA, F. S. 2023. *Uncle Toby's Muesli Bar* [Online]. Fat Secret Australia. Available: https://www.fatsecret.com.au/calories-nutrition/uncle-tobys/muesli-bar/1-bar#:~:text=There%20are%20124%20calories%20in%201%20bar%20of%20Uncle%20Tobys%20Muesli%20Bar. [Accessed 2023].

B, S. 2017. *Junk food companies' advertising budget is 27 TIMES bigger than cash the government uses to promote healthy eating* [Online]. Daily Mail Australia. Available: https://www.dailymail.co.uk/health/article-4968306/Junk-food-ads-spend-27-times-health-scheme.html [Accessed 2023].

BASKIN, K. K., WINDERS, B. R. & OLSON, E. N. 2015. Muscle as a "mediator" of systemic metabolism. *Cell Metab*, 21, 237-248.

BIOLO, G., CEDERHOLM, T. & MUSCARITOLI, M. 2014. Muscle contractile and metabolic dysfunction is a common feature of sarcopenia of aging and chronic diseases: from sarcopenic obesity to cachexia. *Clinical nutrition (Edinburgh, Scotland)*, 33, 737-748.

BROWN, V., ANANTHAPAVAN, J., VEERMAN, L., SACKS, G., LAL, A., PEETERS, A., BACKHOLER, K. & MOODIE, M. 2018. The Potential Cost-Effectiveness and Equity Impacts of Restricting Television Advertising of Unhealthy Food and Beverages to Australian Children. *Nutrients* [Online], 10.

BURRELL, S. 2022. *Your favourite muesli bars ranked by sugar, from highest to lowest.* [Online]. Nine News. Available: https://coach.nine.com.au/diet/muesli-bars-ranked-by-sugar-australia-dietitian-susie-burrell/8b16d655-3e37-4e00-8632-76513d985f5e [Accessed 2023].

CALCOUNT. 2023. *Calories in Muesli Bar, Fruit & Nut* [Online]. Calcount. Available: https://www.caloriecounter.com.au/food/calories-in-muesli-bar-fruit-nut/ [Accessed 2023].

CARRINGTON, K., MORLEY, C., WARREN, S., RYAN, V., BALL, M., CLARKE, J. & VITIS, L. 2021. The impact of COVID-19 pandemic on Australian domestic and family violence services and their clients. *Australian Journal of Social Issues*, 56, 539-558.

CHAMBERS, A. J., ROBERTSON, M. M. & BAKER, N. A. 2019. The effect of sit-stand desks on office worker behavioral and health outcomes: A scoping review. *Appl Ergon*, 78, 37-53.

COMMISSION, E. 2019. *Labelling Nutrition Trans Fats* [Online]. Available: https://food.ec.europa.eu/system/files/2019-04/fs_labelling-nutrition_transfats_swd_ia-pt04.pdf [Accessed 2023].

DIARY, M. N. 2023. *Toast'em Pandan Coconut Bread* [Online]. Available: https://www.mynetdiary.com/food/calories-in-toast-em-pandan-coconut-bread-by-gardenia-slice-28396257-0.html [Accessed 2023].

DIRECTORY, T. Q. C. A. M. 2023. *Queensland's low unemployment continues* [Online]. Available: https://statements.qld.gov.au/statements/97559#:~:text=Queensland's%20trend%20unemployment%20rate%20was,state's%20strong%20labour%20market%20performance [Accessed 2023].

DUPONT, F., LÉGER, P. M., BEGON, M., LECOT, F., SÉNÉCAL, S., LABONTÉ-LEMOYNE, E. & MATHIEU, M. E. 2019. Health and productivity at work: which active workstation for which benefits: a systematic review. *Occup Environ Med,* 76, 281-294.

EDUCATION, D. O. 2023. *Bullying and cyberbullying - preventing and responding* [Online]. Australian Government. Available: https://behaviour.education.qld.gov.au/supporting-student-behaviour/bullying-and-cyberbullying [Accessed 2023].

FARIA, J. 2023. *Ad spend of selected beverage brands in the US 2021* [Online]. Statista. Available: https://www.statista.com/statistics/264985/ad-spend-of-selected-beverage-brands-in-the-us/ [Accessed 2023].

GOVERNMENT, A. 2021. *Australian National Diabetes Strategy* [Online]. Available: https://www.health.gov.au/sites/default/files/documents/2021/11/australian-national-diabetes-strategy-2021-2030_0.pdf [Accessed 2023].

GOVERNMENT, Q. 2018. *Queensland ramps up action on bullying* [Online]. Available: https://statements.qld.gov.au/statements/83941 [Accessed 2023].

GOVERNMENT, Q. 2019. *Queensland Walking Strategy 2019-2029. Walking: for everyone, every day* [Online]. Transport and Main Roads. Available: https://www.tmr.qld.gov.au/-/media/Travelandtransport/Pedestrians-and-walking/Queensland-Walking-Strategy-2019-2029.pdf?la=en [Accessed 2023].

GOVERNMENT, V. 2021. *Cholesterol* [Online]. Better Health Channel. Available: https://www.betterhealth.vic.gov.au/health/conditionsandtreatments/cholesterol [Accessed 2023].

GOVERNMENT, V. 2021. *Triglycerides* [Online]. Better Health Channel. Available: https://www.betterhealth.vic.gov.au/health/conditionsandtreatments/triglycerides [Accessed 2023].

GREENHALGH, E., HURLEY, S, LAL, A. . 2020. *17.4 Economic evaluations of tobacco control interventions* [Online]. Melbourne: Cancer Council Victoria. Available: https://www.tobaccoinaustralia.org.au/chapter-17-economics/17-4-economic-evaluations-of-tobacco-control-interventions [Accessed 2023].

HARRIS J, F.-M. F., PHANEUF L, JENSEN M, CHOI Y, MCCANN M, MANCINI S. 2021. *Fast Food Facts 2021. Fast food advertising: billions in spending, continue high exposure by youth.* [Online]. UConn Rudd Center for Food Policy & Obesity. Available: https://media.ruddcenter.uconn.edu/PDFs/FACTS2021.pdf [Accessed].

HEALTH, D. O. 2019. *National Men's Health Strategy 2020-2030* [Online]. Australian Government. Available: https://www.health.gov.au/sites/default/files/documents/2021/05/national-men-s-health-strategy-2020-2030_0.pdf [Accessed 2023].

HEALTH, Q. 2020. Report of the Chief Health Officer Queensland, the health of Queenslanders 2020.

HEALTH, R. C. F. F. P. 2022. *Rudd Report Executive Summary – Targeted food and beverage advertising to black and Hispanic consumers: 2022 update.* [Online]. University of Connecticut. Available: https://uconnruddcenter.org/wp-content/uploads/sites/2909/2022/11/Rudd-Targeted-Marketing-Report-2022.pdf [Accessed 2023].

HUGHES, K., LOWEY, H., QUIGG, Z. & BELLIS, M. A. 2016. Relationships between adverse childhood experiences and adult mental well-being: results from an English national household survey. *BMC Public Health,* 16**,** 222.

JADAMBAA, A., THOMAS, H. J., SCOTT, J. G., GRAVES, N., BRAIN, D. & PACELLA, R. 2019. Prevalence of traditional bullying and cyberbullying among children and adolescents in Australia: A systematic review and meta-analysis. *Australian & New Zealand Journal of Psychiatry,* 53**,** 878-888.

KIM, H. S., DEMYEN, M. F., MATHEW, J., KOTHARI, N., FEURDEAN, M. & AHLAWAT, S. K. 2017. Obesity, Metabolic Syndrome, and Cardiovascular Risk in Gluten-Free Followers Without Celiac Disease in the United States: Results from the National Health and Nutrition Examination Survey 2009-2014. *Dig Dis Sci,* 62**,** 2440-2448.

KING, C. 2023. *Carman's Classic Fruit & Nut Muesli Bar* [Online]. Calorie King. Available: https://www.calorieking.com/au/en/foods/f/calories-in-bars-classic-fruit-nut-muesli-bar/TVE11n-eTSP22Iqb_4GrGbQ [Accessed 2023].

KPMG. 2022. *Shifting the dial on vegetable consumption – Rebuilding healthy families in a COVID-19 affected and disrupted Australia* [Online]. Available: https://static1.squarespace.com/static/5ddca44a3ac7644d97d9757a/t/633e2e9e396cdd49c-cfa3ee9/1665019635620/FVC+Report_Final_041022.pdf [Accessed].

LEE, A. J., PATAY, D., HERRON, L.-M., TAN, R. C., NICOLL, E., FREDERICKS, B. & LEWIS, M. 2021. Affordability of Heathy, Equitable and More Sustainable Diets in Low-Income Households in Brisbane before and during the COVID-19 Pandemic. *Nutrients* [Online], 13.

LOWE, I. 2023. *Why Australia needs to change its thinking on growing the economy* [Online]. Sydney Morning Herald. Available: https://www.smh.com.au/environment/sustainability/why-australia-needs-to-change-its-thinking-on-growing-the-economy-20230404-p5cy04.html [Accessed 2023].

MANAGER, C. 2023. *Carbs in Liberated Coconut Bread* [Online]. Wombat Apps. Available: https://www.carbmanager.com/food-detail/md:131d518b51a40fde7a6d08a25203ceb4/coconut-[Accessed 2023].

MÁRMOL-SOLER, C., MATIAS, S., MIRANDA, J., LARRETXI, I., FERNÁNDEZ-GIL, M. D. P., BUSTAMANTE, M., CHURRUCA, I., MARTÍNEZ, O. & SIMÓN, E. 2022. Gluten-Free Products: Do We Need to Update Our Knowledge? *Foods,* 11.

MCGREGOR, R. A. & POPPITT, S. D. 2013. Milk protein for improved metabolic health: a review of the evidence. *Nutr Metab (Lond),* 10, 46.

MEDICINE, N. L. O. 2023. *Cholesterol testing and results* [Online]. Available: https://medlineplus.gov/ency/patientinstructions/000386.htm [Accessed 2023].

MINGES, K. E., CHAO, A. M., IRWIN, M. L., OWEN, N., PARK, C., WHITTEMORE, R. & SALMON, J. 2016. Classroom Standing Desks and Sedentary Behavior: A Systematic Review. *Pediatrics,* 137, e20153087.

MINNESOTA, U. O. 2022. *What is the difference between fats and oils?* [Online]. Available: https://reallifegoodfood.umn.edu/eat/nutrition/myplate/fats-and-oils [Accessed 2023].

MORLEY, C., CARRINGTON, K., RYAN, V., WARREN, S., CLARKE, J., BALL, M. & VITIS, L. 2021. Locked Down with the Perpetrator: The Hidden Impacts of COVID-19 on Domestic and Family Violence in Australia. *International Journal for Crime, Justice and Social Democracy,* 10, 204-222.

MUCH, E. T. 2023. *Coconut Bread* [Online]. Available: https://www.eatthismuch.com/food/nutrition/coconut-bread,2443539/ [Accessed 2023].

MUCH, E. T. 2023. *Muesli Bar - Oats and Seeds Woolworths* [Online]. Eat This Much. Available: https://www.eatthismuch.com/food/nutrition/muesli-bar,164039/ [Accessed 2023].

NATALIE BUTLER, Y. B. 2023. *How many calories should I eat a day?* [Online]. Medical News Today. Available: https://www.medicalnewstoday.com/articles/245588 [Accessed 2023].

NUTRITIONIX. 2023. *Coconut Bread - 1 piece* [Online]. A Syndigo Company. Available: https://www.nutritionix.com/i/nutritionix/coconut-bread-1-piece/5909e48a3a2b319e22f25df3 [Accessed 2023].

OBESITY, W. 2022. *Weight Stigma* [Online]. Available: https://www.worldobesity.org/what-we-do/our-policy-priorities/weight-stigma [Accessed 2023].

OFFICE, Q. G. S. S. 2018. *Queensland Government population projects* [Online]. Queensland Treasury. Available: https://www.qgso.qld.gov.au/issues/2671/qld-government-population-projections-2018-edn.pdf [Accessed 2023].

OFFICE, Q. G. S. S. 2021. *COVID-19 and DFV assault offence trends, March–September 2020.* [Online]. Queensland Treasury. Available: https://www.qgso.qld.gov.au/issues/11116/covid-19-dfv-assault-offence-trends-march-september-2020.pdf [Accessed 2023].

OLSHANSKY, S. J., PASSARO, D. J., HERSHOW, R. C., LAYDEN, J., CARNES, B. A., BRODY, J., HAYFLICK, L., BUTLER, R. N., ALLISON, D. B. & LUDWIG, D. S. 2005. A potential decline in life expectancy in the United States in the 21st century. *N Engl J Med,* 352**,** 1138-45.

ORGANISATION, W. H. 2023. *Constitution* [Online]. WHO. Available: https://www.who.int/about/governance/constitution [Accessed 2023].

ORQUIN, J. L. & SCHOLDERER, J. 2015. Consumer judgments of explicit and implied health claims on foods: Misguided but not misled. *Food Policy,* 51**,** 144-157.

PASE, M. P., GRIMA, N., COCKERELL, R. & PIPINGAS, A. 2015. Habitual intake of fruit juice predicts central blood pressure. *Appetite,* 84**,** 68-72.

PAYNE, J. L., MORGAN, A. & PIQUERO, A. R. 2022. COV-

ID-19 and social distancing measures in Queensland, Australia, are associated with short-term decreases in recorded violent crime. *Journal of Experimental Criminology,* 18**,** 89-113.

PROFESSOR AMANDA LEE, L.-M. H., PROFESSOR BRONWYN FREDERICKS. 7 April 2022 2022. As we face a "perfect storm" for food security, here are some solutions. Available from: https://medicine.uq.edu.au/blog/2022/04/we-face-%E2%80%9Cperfect-storm%E2%80%9D-food-security-here-are-some-solutions 2023].

PRONK, N. P. 2019. Public health, business, and the shared value of workforce health and wellbeing. *Lancet Public Health,* 4**,** e323.

PUHL, R. & SUH, Y. 2015. Health Consequences of Weight Stigma: Implications for Obesity Prevention and Treatment. *Current Obesity Reports,* 4**,** 182-190.

QUEENSLAND, H. A. W. 2020. *Opinion Articles* [Online]. Brisbane, Queensland, Australia: Queensland Government. Available: https://hw.qld.gov.au/blog/category/opinion/ [Accessed 2023].

QUEENSLAND, H. A. W. 2021. *Obesity and COVID-19: It's time to double down* [Online]. Available: https://hw.qld.gov.au/blog/obesity-and-covid-19-its-time-to-double-down/ [Accessed 2023].

RAVESTEIJN, B., VAN KIPPERSLUIS, H. & VAN DOORSLAER, E. 2013. The contribution of occupation to health inequality. *Res Econ Inequal,* 21**,** 311-332.

RESEARCH, C. S. A. I. 2022. *Cholesterol Facts* [Online]. CSIRO. Available: https://www.csiro.au/en/research/health-medical/nutrition/cholesterol-facts#:~:text=Total%20Cholesterol%3A%20%3C4.0%20mmol%2F,)%3A%20%3C%202.0%20mmol%2FL [Accessed 2023].

SAINI, R. K., PRASAD, P., SREEDHAR, R. V., AKHILENDER NAIDU, K., SHANG, X. & KEUM, Y.-S. 2021. Omega−3 Polyunsaturated Fatty Acids (PUFAs): Emerging Plant and Microbial Sources, Oxidative Stability, Bioavailability, and Health Benefits—A Review. *Antioxidants* [Online], 10.

SERVICE, Q. C. O. S. 2020. *COVID-19 impacts on Queenslanders. The unfolding impacts of COVID-19 and how they are distributed among different people.* [Online]. Available: https://www.qcoss.org.au/wp-content/uploads/2021/02/QCOSS-Queensland-Impacts-COVID-19.pdf [Accessed 2023].

SETTLE, P. J., CAMERON, A. J. & THORNTON, L. E. 2014. Socioeconomic differences in outdoor food advertising at public transit stops across Melbourne suburbs. *Australian and New Zealand Journal of Public Health,* 38**,** 414-418.

SHREFFLER, J., PETREY, J. & HUECKER, M. 2020. The Impact of COVID-19 on Healthcare Worker Wellness: A Scoping Review. *West J Emerg Med,* 21**,** 1059-1066.

STATISTICS, A. B. O. 2017-18. *Diabetes* [Online]. ABS. Available: https://www.abs.gov.au/statistics/health/health-conditions-and-risks/diabetes/2017-18#cite-window1 [Accessed 2023].

STATISTICS, A. B. O. 2017-18. *Health conditions and risks - Overweight and obesity* [Online]. ABS. Available: https://www.abs.gov.au/statistics/health/health-conditions-and-risks/overweight-and-obesity/latest-release#cite-window2 [Accessed 2023].

STATISTICS, A. B. O. 2020-21. *Diabetes* [Online]. ABS. Available: https://www.abs.gov.au/statistics/health/health-conditions-and-risks/diabetes/latest-release [Accessed 2023].

STATISTICS, A. B. O. 2022. *A caring nation – 15 per cent of Australia's workforce in Health Care and Social Assistance industry* [Online]. ABS. Available: https://www.abs.gov.au/media-centre/media-releases/caring-nation-15-cent-australias-workforce-health-care-and-social-assistance-industry [Accessed 2023].

TAM, B. T., MORAIS, J. A. & SANTOSA, S. 2020. Obesity and ageing: Two sides of the same coin. *Obesity Reviews,* 21, e12991.

TANVEER, M. & AHMED, A. 2019. Non-Celiac Gluten Sensitivity: A Systematic Review. *J Coll Physicians Surg Pak,* 29, 51-57.

THOMPSON C, M. D., BIRD S 2022. Evaluation of the Improving Social Connectedness of Older

Australians project pilot: Informing future policy considerations. *In:* CENTRE FOR HEALTH SERVICE DEVELOPMENT & INSTITUTE, A. H. S. R. (eds.). University of Wollongong.

TOMIYAMA, A. J., CARR, D., GRANBERG, E. M., MAJOR, B., ROBINSON, E., SUTIN, A. R. & BREWIS, A. 2018. How and why weight stigma drives the obesity 'epidemic' and harms health. *BMC Med,* 16, 123.

TREASURY, Q. 2023. *Economy, Labour and Employment (State)* [Online]. Queensland Government Statistician's Office. Available: https://www.qgso.qld.gov.au/statistics/theme/economy/labour-employment/state [Accessed 2023].

TREASURY, Q. 2023. *Queensland Government Statistician's Office – Labour and employment.* [Online]. Queensland Government. Available: https://www.qgso.qld.gov.au/statistics/theme/economy/labour-employment/state [Accessed 2023].

UNIVERSITY, H. 2023. *Types of Fat* [Online]. School of Public Health. Available: https://www.hsph.harvard.edu/nutritionsource/what-should-you-eat/fats-and-cholesterol/types-of-fat/ [Accessed 2023].

VARADY, K. A., CIENFUEGOS, S., EZPELETA, M. & GABEL, K. 2021. Cardiometabolic Benefits of Intermittent Fasting. *Annual Review of Nutrition,* 41, 333-361.

WELFARE, A. I. O. H. A. 2017. *Aging and welfare* [Online]. AIHW. Available: https://www.aihw.gov.au/getmedia/d18a1d2b-692c-42bf-81e2-47cd54c51e8d/aihw-australias-welfare-2017-chapter5-1.pdf.aspx [Accessed 2023].

WELFARE, A. I. O. H. A. 2018. *New report shows long-term disadvantage for Australia's Stolen Generations* [Online]. AIHW. Available: https://www.aihw.gov.au/news-media/media-releases/2018/august/new-report-shows-long-term-disadvantage-for-austra [Accessed 2023].

WELFARE, A. I. O. H. A. 2020. *Indicators for the Australian National Diabetes Strategy 2016–2020: data update* [Online]. Australian Government. Available: https://www.aihw.gov.au/reports/diabetes/diabetes-indicators-strategy-2016-2020/contents/goal-1-prevent-people-developing-type-2-diabetes/1-7-total-energy-intake-from-saturated-fatty-acids [Accessed 2023].

WELFARE, A. I. O. H. A. 2021. *Social isolation and loneliness* [Online]. AIHW. Available: https://www.aihw.gov.au/reports/australias-welfare/social-isolation-and-loneliness-covid-pandemic [Accessed 2023].

References

WELFARE, A. I. O. H. A. 2022. *Australia's Health 2022: in brief* [Online]. Available: https://www.aihw.gov.au/getmedia/c6c5d-da9-4020-43b0-8ed6-a567cd660eaa/aihw-aus-241.pdf.aspx?in-line=true [Accessed Australia's health series number 18].

WELFARE, A. I. O. H. A. 2022. *Australia's health 2022 – data insights: Changes in the health of Australians during the COV-ID-19 period.* [Online]. Available: https://www.aihw.gov.au/get-media/cb5f5bbb-df0b-4a1c-9796-25ea2e94e447/aihw-aus-240_Chapter_2.pdf.aspx [Accessed 2 Australia's Health 2022].

WELFARE, A. I. O. H. A. 2022. *Australia's health 2022, data insights: Mental health of young Australians* [Online]. Available: https://www.aihw.gov.au/getmedia/ba6da461-a046-44ac-9a7f-29d08a2bea9f/aihw-aus-240_Chapter_8.pdf.aspx [Accessed 8].

WELFARE, A. I. O. H. A. 2022. *Bullying* [Online]. AIHW. Available: https://www.aihw.gov.au/reports/children-youth/australi-as-children/contents/justice-and-safety/bullying [Accessed 2023].

WELFARE, A. I. O. H. A. 2022. *Chronic conditions and multi-morbidity* [Online]. AIHW. Available: https://www.aihw.gov.au/reports/australias-health/chronic-conditions-and-multimorbidity [Accessed 2023].

WELFARE, A. I. O. H. A. 2022. *Disease expenditure in Austral-ia 2019-20* [Online]. AIHW. Available: https://www.aihw.gov.au/getmedia/f1a20cd3-c24c-45e4-ae00-9a6f9c95903c/Disease-ex-penditure-in-Australia-2019-20.pdf.aspx?inline=true [Accessed 2023].

WELFARE, A. I. O. H. A. 2022. *Mental Health Services in Australia: Stress and Trauma* [Online]. AIHW. Available: https://www.aihw.gov.au/reports/mental-health-services/stress-and-trau-ma [Accessed 2023].

WELFARE, A. I. O. H. A. 2022. *Mental health: prevalence and impact* [Online]. Australian Government. Available: https://www.aihw.gov.au/reports/mental-health-services/mental-health [Accessed 2023].

WELFARE, A. I. O. H. A. 2023. *Chronic Disease* [Online]. AIHW. Available: https://www.aihw.gov.au/reports-data/health-conditions-disability-deaths/chronic-disease/overview [Accessed 2023].

WORKS, D. O. H. A. P. 2023. *Queensland Housing Profiles – dwelling and household characteristics, Queensland* [Online]. Queensland Government. Available: https://statistics.qgso.qld.gov.au/profiles/hpw/housing/pdf/45G-DHLQXHD202HNVA6QGE217OEO692F1K3Q56UO94R-2P2R7JK0VF7T6SJ4JQO5Z2HT58BC5FXT6GT8R8EJLH-VMU48AWUZNBLK8YE3CYHT1V11X1YO58JRT6P322B-0G0I/hpw-housing-profiles#view=fit&pagemode=bookmarks [Accessed 2023].

ZACHARIAS, K. D., HUNDAL, N., KUMAR, S., SHIGEMATSU, L. M. R., BAHL, D. & WIPFLI, H. 2019. Corporate Wellness Programs: Promoting a Healthy Workforce. *In:* WITHERS, M. & MCCOOL, J. (eds.) *Global Health Leadership: Case Studies From the Asia-Pacific.* Cham: Springer International Publishing.

ZEALAND, G. O. N. 2020. *Wellbeing Budget 2020: Rebuilding Together* [Online]. Government of New Zealand. Available: https://www.treasury.govt.nz/publications/wellbeing-budget/wellbeing-budget-2020#from-the-prime-minister [Accessed 2023].